SUPER
FOODS
for
PREGNANCY

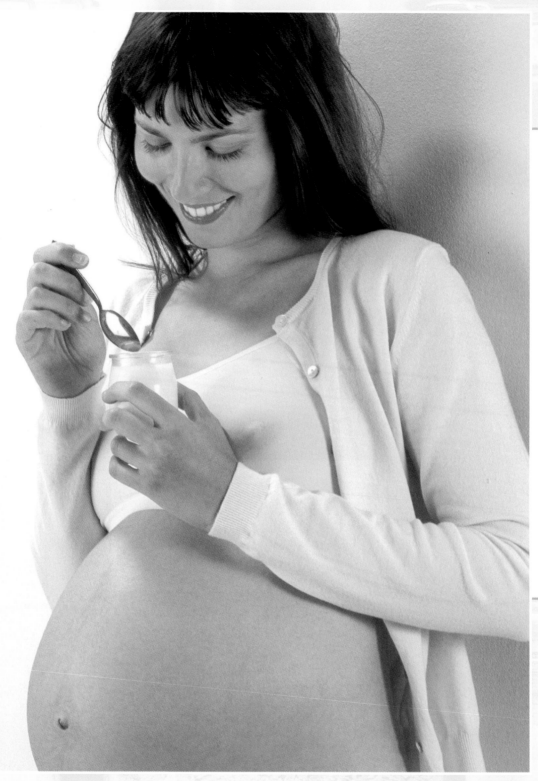

SUPER FOODS
for
PREGNANCY

**DELICIOUS WAYS TO MEET YOUR
KEY DIETARY REQUIREMENTS**

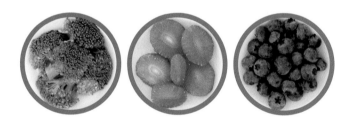

SUSANNAH MARRIOTT

hamlyn

For Berry and her garden

An Hachette UK company
www.hachette.co.uk

First published in Great Britain in 2011 by
Carroll & Brown Publishers Limited

This second edition published in 2015 by
Hamlyn, a division of
Octopus Publishing Group Ltd
Carmelite House
50 Victoria Embankment
London, EC4Y 0DZ
www.octopusbooksusa.com

Copyright © Octopus Publishing Group Ltd
2011, 2015
Text copyright © Susannah Marriott
2011, 2015

Distributed in the US by
Hachette Book Group
1290 Avenue of the Americas, 4th and
5th Floors, New York, NY 10020

Distributed in Canada by
Canadian Manda Group
664 Annette Street, Toronto, Ontario,
Canada M6S 2C8

ISBN 978-0-600-63160-6

Printed and bound in China

10 9 8 7 6 5 4 3 2 1

Art Director Chrissie Lloyd
Managing Art Editor Emily Cook
Photography Jules Selmes, David Murray
Editorial Assistance Idroma Montgomery

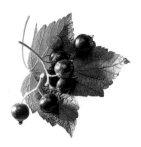

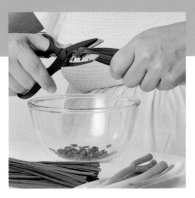

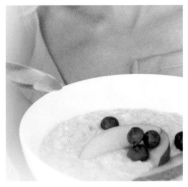

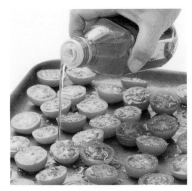

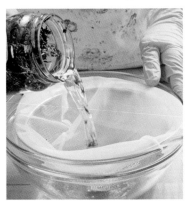

CONTENTS

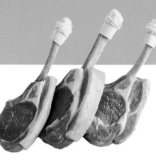

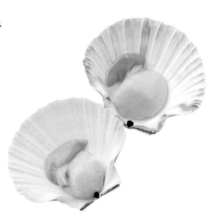

INTRODUCTION

There is no better time in life to become obsessed with food and how it grows than when you are pregnant. Eating good, seasonal food will provide you with almost everything you need to nourish your changing body and nurture your growing baby. This book focuses on choosing or growing the best vegetables, fruit, and herbs and sourcing great meat, fish, dairy produce, and whole grains. Maximum nutrition during pregnancy is a result of eating a wide variety of foods from these groups most days.

Growing your own food (entries marked with plant symbol)—even just a pot of herbs on a windowsill—fulfills an instinctive need to provide your baby with the best possible nourishment. A spot of gardening also supplies exactly what pregnancy demands: gentle, regular exercise, lots of vitamin D from sunlight to boost your calcium supplies, the freshest produce, and an opportunity to "nest" outdoors. Growing food also is a form of creativity and self-expression that helps you to embrace your home, particularly if you have previously spent long hours at work. Like any craft, it brings the satisfaction of creating something beautiful. You don't need a formal garden—you can grow edible plants in pots and window boxes, on balconies and windowsills and vertically, too, trained up walls and tumbling from hanging baskets. Growing stuff roots you in the soil and the place you live like nothing else, linking you to its unique weather, food traditions, heritage varieties, and plant lore. In time, you can pass that knowledge on to your children.

Along with growing food, eating local puts you in touch with the seasons' bounty—such as spring's early sweet peas, which can be popped straight into your mouth, and the long anticipated harvest pumpkin watched all summer as its belly swelled with promise. Home-grown and locally sold produce ensures extra-ripe food and more diverse, delicate crops that can't cope with long journeys. If you've always shopped at supermarkets, this can be a revelation. It teaches patience and trust in the processes of growth and regeneration in the natural world, even as they are happening inside you. Buying local produce helps to protect the food chain and environment for our children and sustains the

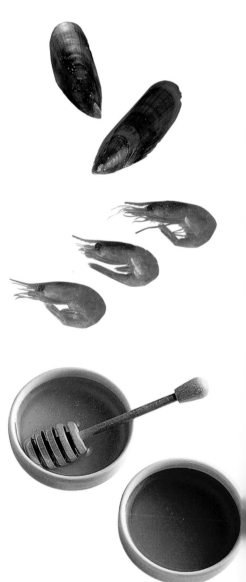

neighboring economy: if we eat what the land around us grows, we safeguard centuries of tradition, employment, and precious views for future generations. Gardening and mothering both encourage us to think into the future and about the past. In this book I encourage you to think about others, too, by involving your family, neighbors, and friends in your quest to eat better, thereby nurturing an extended family of gardeners.

Planting information will be given wherever you see this symbol.

The stages of pregnancy uncannily reflect the seasons of growth in the natural world, and wherever you are in your pregnancy and the growing season, just thinking about sowing, ripening, and harvest will help you to adjust to the changes in your body. Being in touch with nature is key to not only maintaining physical well-being but also for peace of mind. It gives us "vitamin G" or green space. The Dutch public health expert Peter Groenewegen describes this as the key to better physical health, emotional well-being, and a sense of security in the place we call home. Spending time among greenery is known to be of special help during periods of anxiety and change, helping individuals to rebalance fluctuating moods and regain a measure of control.

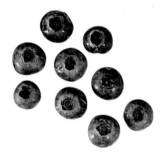

My appetite grew with my pregnancies, but my love of gardening dwindled; with my first pregnancy, simply stepping into the garden would bring on overwhelming feelings of nausea. So, if you don't feel like growing stuff, don't; you can source all this produce at the farmers' market or farm gate, or have boxes of fish, meat, or seasonal vegetables delivered direct to your doorstep. We have every right to be lazy when our bodies are doing so much work behind the scenes.

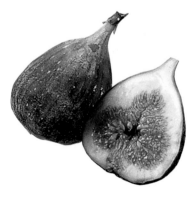

Even if you feel super-lazy, do take the opportunity to turn a little of the available delicious fresh produce into some of the seasonal dishes described at the end of this book. The recipes have been created especially for their nutritional benefits in pregnancy—and beyond—as well as trying the quick-and-easy suggestions. They suit infant-centered weaning and I hope they encourage you to sit around the table as a family enjoying the miracle of growth in all its forms.

SUPER NUTRIENTS

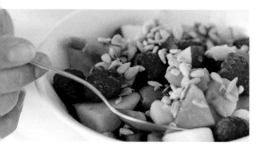

Good food keeps us feeling fit and energized during pregnancy. In one study, women who ate a diet based on fish, low-fat meat and dairy foods, healthy oils, whole grains, and plenty of fruit, vegetables, and legumes reduced their chance of delivering early by 90 percent. The nutrients we need are absorbed most effectively when we eat a wide variety of foods daily, rather than by taking supplements alone. Here is a guide to the essentials you need to keep your body working well, your energy levels high, and your emotions balanced—and to make sure your baby gets the best possible start in life.

MUST-HAVE VITAMINS

VITAMIN A

This comes from retinol in animal produce and beta-carotene in plant foods. It is critical during intense periods of cell growth in pregnancy, particularly in the first and last trimesters, when it protects against cell mutation and aids eye and lung development. Low levels reduce your immune function, making infections more likely. A good intake is said to help guard against stretch marks, but too much retinol can harm the developing fetus (see page 121).
Food sources: *milk, butter, cheese, eggs, chicken, oily fish, beet, peas, beans, asparagus, broccoli, spinach, winter squash, carrots, lettuce, dandelion leaves, apricots.*

B VITAMINS

Certain ones are vital for energy production (B_1 thiamin, B_2 riboflavin, and B_3 niacin) and for a baby's developing nervous system, brain, red blood cells, and muscles. Others promote endurance and regulate your stress hormones (B_6 pyridoxine and B_{12} cobalamin). You need more B_1 and B_2 during pregnancy to maintain your energy reserves and nerve and muscle function, plus B_2 to promote iron absorption. Women who have greater amounts of B_3 seem to give birth to longer babies

with higher birthweights and larger head circumference, all signs of good health. A good intake of B_6 seems to be associated with reduced pregnancy nausea. If you are vegetarian or vegan, ask your doctor whether you need a B_{12} supplement while pregnant and breastfeeding, since a deficiency in infants is linked with neurological damage.
Food sources: *red meat, clams, oily fish, seaweed, eggs, milk, yogurt, hard cheese, chicken, sunflower seeds, whole grains, almonds, bananas, avocados.*

FOLATE

This is the essential pregnancy B vitamin. You need double the normal amount now and should take

---

DAILY DIET

Aim for the following each day:

2–3 servings of meat, fish, nuts, and legumes
2–3 servings of green leafy vegetables
3 servings of fruit and other vegetables
3 servings of whole grains
3–4 servings of dairy produce

---

a supplement of 400 mcg folic acid (the synthetic form) daily from the time you start thinking about pregnancy until the end of the first trimester, when your baby's spinal cord is forming. Taking folic acid significantly lowers a baby's risk of neural tube defects (such as spina bifida). Once you find out you are pregnant it can be too late to make a difference. Folate helps in the formation of red blood cells and DNA. In some studies, women who take folic acid supplements suffer fewer infections in pregnancy and have babies with higher birth weights and a better Apgar score (this assesses the health of a newborn). Lack of folic acid is the world's most common vitamin deficiency. You may need a higher dose of folic acid (5 mg daily) if you have diabetes or had neural tube problems in a previous pregnancy—talk to your doctor.
Food sources: *spinach, broccoli, peas, asparagus, lentils, cabbage, beets, beans, winter squash, parsnips, lettuce, mustard greens, blackberries, pomegranates, avocados, chickpeas, lentils, whole grains, eggs, papayas, bananas.*

VITAMIN C

This is good for the production of new tissue, for keeping the immune system strong, and aiding iron absorption. A good supply of this vitamin may help to prevent bleeding gums, reduce pregnancy nausea, and lessen the risk of pre-eclampsia. In a University of North Carolina study, lack of vitamin C seemed to increase the risk of the premature rupture of membranes, a leading cause of premature birth. To maximize absorption, cook with a little olive oil.

Food sources: *black currants, kiwi, guava, grapefruit, cantaloupe melon, oranges, papaya, sweet peppers, strawberries, blackberries, raspberries, Brussels sprouts, tomatoes, broccoli, spinach, winter squash, kale, asparagus, sweet potatoes, peas, sauerkraut.*

VITAMIN D

This is vital for your baby's developing teeth and bones and for promoting good levels of calcium and phosphate for your own bones and teeth. We get most of our vitamin D from sunlight (expose your skin for 15–20 minutes a day if you can), but take a daily supplement of 10 mcg, especially if you have darker skin, don't go outside much, or prefer to cover up while outdoors.

Food sources: *oily fish, red meat, egg yolk, milk, butter.*

VITAMIN K

Essential for strong bones since it traps calcium in the bones, it may also help to ease pregnancy nausea. Vitamin K aids blood clotting, preventing excessive bleeding, so a good dietary intake may be helpful in the run-up to childbirth. An injection of vitamin K is routinely given to newborns to prevent bleeding problems.

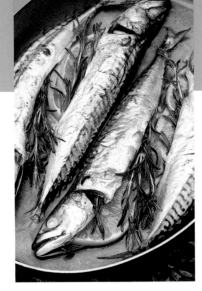

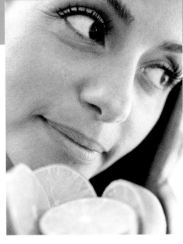

Food sources: *kale, spinach, mustard greens, Brussels sprouts, broccoli, dandelion leaves, lettuce, asparagus.*

MUST-HAVE MINERALS

CALCIUM

Our bodies become more efficient at absorbing this important bone-building mineral from food from the second trimester onward and while breastfeeding. As well as building your baby's teeth and bones, calcium helps the development of nerves and muscles. Many of us are calcium-deficient (the average woman only gets three-quarters of what she needs), and if your baby doesn't receive enough calcium from your diet, he or she will "borrow" it from your bones, leading to an increased risk of osteoporosis later in life. A low dietary intake has been associated with a greater risk of pre-eclampsia and with muscle cramps; it is also said to increase the pain of labor. An adequate supply of calcium may lower the risk of delivering early and pregnancy-related high blood pressure.

Calcium is especially bone-protecting when combined with vitamins C and K and magnesium (a combination found in spinach) and with vitamin D (from 15–20 minutes' daily exposure to sunlight). If you do not eat dairy produce or are in your teens, talk to your doctor about calcium supplements.

Food sources: *yogurt, cheese, milk, small fish with edible bones, almonds, sesame seeds, broccoli, peas, beans, kale, dandelion leaves, cabbage, spinach, beet leaves.*

IRON

Although the body becomes more efficient at absorbing iron from food as pregnancy progresses, it's quite common to begin pregnancy deficient in this important mineral, which helps muscles to develop, is vital for the manufacture of red blood cells, and guards against anemia (a deficiency of the red blood cells that carry oxygen and nutrients around the body and to your baby). Having a good amount of iron protects against early delivery and low birthweight. If you are in your teens, have had pregnancies in quick succession, or are planning a home birth, talk to your doctor about a supplement.

Vitamin C aids the body's uptake of iron, whereas tea and coffee hinder absorption, so accompany

meals with fruit or fruit juice.
Food sources: *red meat, poultry (the darker meat), small fish with edible bones, seafood, cabbage, nettles, broccoli, spinach, beets, peas, beans, asparagus, whole grains, legumes.*

COPPER

This trace mineral helps to build a baby's heart and circulatory system, while repairing your own tissues. It is especially important in the third trimester, since your baby is born with four times the amount of copper as an adult, relying on it for many metabolic functions, including those of the heart and immune system. When copper occurs naturally with iron, as in spinach, it promotes the uptake of iron.
Food sources: *hazelnuts, peas, beans, whole grains, oysters, cocoa, spinach, beets, asparagus.*

MAGNESIUM

Required for the development of healthy bones, cells, nerve function, and blood clotting, this mineral protects cardiovascular health and may help in lowering high blood pressure. It helps muscles to relax, easing leg cramps, migraines, and insomnia. It is associated with reducing pregnancy nausea and women with a good intake seem to have a lessened risk of early delivery and low-birthweight babies. It also promotes calcium absorption.
Food sources: *pumpkin and sunflower seeds, milk, almonds, brown rice, broccoli, spinach, beets, peas, beans, whole grains.*

ZINC

This mineral is required by your baby's developing nervous system and bones and supports immune function. During pregnancy, zinc levels dip and low levels have been associated with low-birthweight babies and an increased risk of neural tube defects. If you are

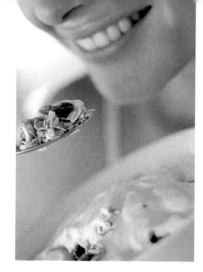

prescribed an iron supplement, increase the number of zinc-rich foods in your diet.
Food sources: *red meat, pumpkin seeds, poultry, seafood, whole grains.*

SELENIUM

During pregnancy you need slightly more of this powerful antioxidant, which safeguards cell development. Low levels may be linked with miscarriage and an increased risk of pre-eclampsia.
Food sources: *Brazil nuts, walnuts, almonds, whole grains, fish, seafood, poultry, red meat, eggs, garlic.*

POTASSIUM

This mineral is essential for good fluid balance, to support the rise in blood volume, for energy-release, and nerve and muscle impulses. If you suffer from leg cramps, try increasing your dietary intake. Also increase your intake while breastfeeding.
Food sources: *potatoes, beets, beans, lentils, clams, fish, winter squash, carrots, figs, prunes, apricots, avocados, Jerusalem artichokes, yogurt, bananas.*

MANGANESE

This important mineral helps to build strong bones, protect cells from damage, and boost energy

production, especially when combined with copper.
Food sources: *whole grains, chickpeas, lentils, hazelnuts, walnuts, almonds, kale, spinach, beans, raspberries, strawberries, garlic.*

CHROMIUM

This trace mineral helps to build protein in a baby's developing tissues. Because it balances levels of glucose in the body, it is especially important if you have diabetes or develop gestational diabetes. It can be depleted by a diet high in refined sugar and processed foods.
Food sources: *beef, poultry, eggs, oysters, spinach, peanut butter, lettuce, apples, onions, bananas.*

PHOSPHORUS

This mineral works with calcium to build strong bones and teeth both in you and your baby. Phosphorus is also required for the growth and repair of tissue and cells, and is important for well-functioning muscles, nerves, kidneys, and heart. It regulates energy use and can be effective in reducing pain after a period of exertion.
Food sources: *yogurt, milk, cheese, oily fish, poultry, lentils, eggs, peas, beans, almonds, whole wheat, garlic.*

MORE FOOD MUST-HAVES

PROTEIN

The amino acids that make up protein form the building blocks of every cell and tissue in your baby's body and supply you with the means of maintaining and repairing your own cells, organs, and tissue. Protein-rich foods are a good source of vitamins and minerals, too. A typical Western diet tends to give us all the protein we need.

The most "complete" form of protein is found in animal foods, which contain all the essential amino acids the human body requires. If you don't eat meat, combining different plant proteins through the day will give you the balance of amino acids you need.

Food sources: *eggs, red meat, fish, poultry, seafood, milk, cheese, oats, nuts and seeds, lentils, whole grains, peas, chickpeas, beans, yogurt.*

CHOLINE

This is an essential amino acid required for the healthy development of a baby's brain and memory. Deficiency increases the risk of neural tube defects, especially if you lack folate. Most of us are deficient in choline, and need to add more to our diet during pregnancy and breastfeeding. Without adequate choline we can become deficient in folate, too.

Food sources: *egg yolk, poultry, red meat, shrimp, potatoes, lentils, cauliflower, oats, sesame seeds.*

FIBER

Eating some insoluble dietary fiber every day—found in whole wheat and vegetables—can help to prevent and ease constipation. Soluble fiber in oats, legumes, and fruit helps you to feel fuller for longer and keeps blood-sugar levels stable while enhancing the immune system's reaction to bacterial infection. A fiber-rich diet also helps to maintain healthy digestive tract flora. The form of plant fiber known as fructooligosaccharide (FOS) is particularly effective at promoting the growth of beneficial lactobacilli and bifidobacteria in the digestive system.

Sources: *whole grains, lentils, broccoli, cabbage, spinach, peas, beans, asparagus, parsnips, carrots, onions, blackberries, apples.*

OMEGA-3 FATTY ACIDS

Docosahexaenoic acid (DHA) is the fatty acid vital for the development of a baby's brain, eyes, and nervous system, and for ensuring heart health in later life. It is particularly important in the third trimester, when growth of fetal brain tissue is especially rapid, and during breast-feeding. In clinical trials, mothers with higher levels of omega-3 fatty acids had a significantly reduced risk of premature delivery; they also seemed to have babies with higher birthweights and cognitive development scores in early childhood. DHA may be useful in maintaining emotional balance after birth and speeding up postnatal recovery, and may affect infant sleep patterns for the better. The typical Western diet is alarmingly low in DHA and pregnancy additionally (particularly with twins or more) depletes reserves. One study says that we only consume 20 percent of what we need in pregnancy.

Eating too many sources of omega-6 fatty acids (found in processed foods) can throw out a healthy balance of omega-3 fatty acids (see page 121). Alpha-linolenic acid (ALA) from plant sources converts to DHA in the body, but not very well.

Food sources: *DHA from oily coldwater fish such as salmon, mackerel, tuna, herring, anchovies, algae, seaweed; ALA from flax seeds and oil, walnuts, pumpkin seeds.*

PHYTONUTRIENTS

These biologically active components of plants supply a plant's unique flavor and color and benefit our health. The largest category is made up of polyphenols, which are responsible, for example, for the color of blueberries, the flavor of olives, and the pungency of onions. They have a powerful antioxidant action, protecting against cell damage, and are also anti-inflammatory, antibacterial and antiviral and can relax the blood vessels. More research needs to be done into the role of phytonutrients in pregnancy, but a paper in the *Journal of the American Nutraceutical Association* suggested that a diet rich in phytonutrients could decrease pregnancy complications, resulting in fewer cesarean deliveries, premature births, and pre-eclampsia.

Make sure you eat some yellow, red, purple, and green vegetables and fruit daily to ensure a good intake of phytonutrients.

Food sources: *apples, oranges, pineapples, cranberries, peaches, acerola, cherries, papayas, carrots, parsley, beets, kale, broccoli, cabbage, spinach, and tomatoes.*

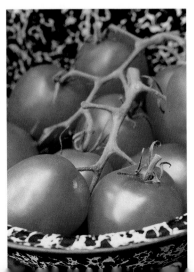

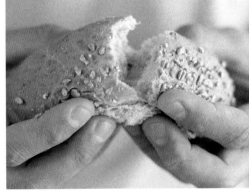

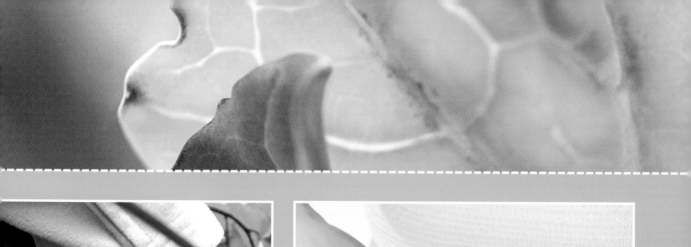
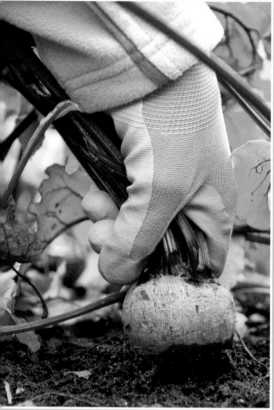
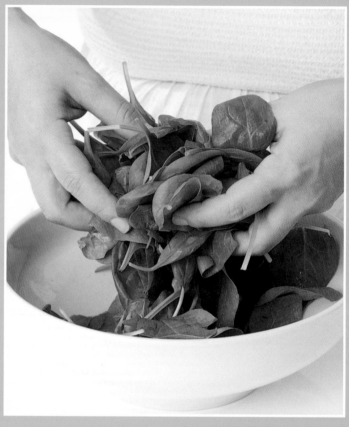
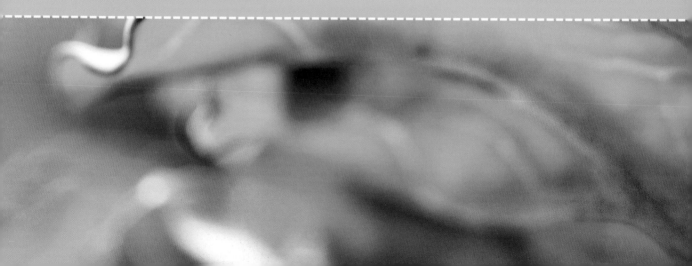

GOODNESS FROM THE GARDEN

These wonder foods offer plenty of nutrients to nourish your growing baby and ease various complaints such as morning sickness while also being a treat for your taste buds. Enthusiastic gardeners might like to raise a few of these must-have vegetables and fruits at home. If you lack the patience to grow your own from seed, or it sounds like too much work, the farmers' market is the place to go for young plants. They also are much more likely to sell produce with home-grown flavor and varieties too delicate or ripe for the supermarket shelves.

BROCCOLI · CABBAGE · BRUSSELS SPROUTS · KALE · SPINACH · SWISS CHARD · BEETS
PEAS · SNOW PEAS · FAVA BEANS · GREEN BEANS · RUNNER BEANS · ASPARAGUS
WINTER SQUASH · POTATOES · PARSNIPS · CARROTS · GINGER · BLACK CURRANTS
RASPBERRIES · SUMMER SALADS · MUSTARD GREENS · TOMATOES · GARLIC
SCALLIONS · CHIVES · LEMONS · STRAWBERRIES · BLUEBERRIES

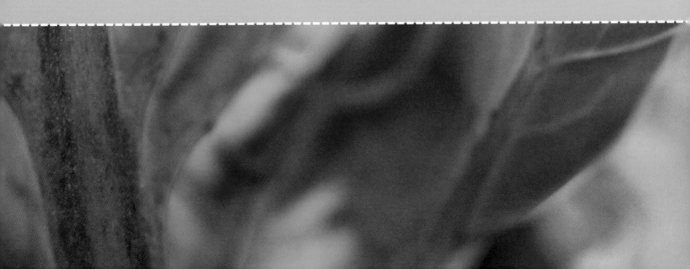

BROCCOLI

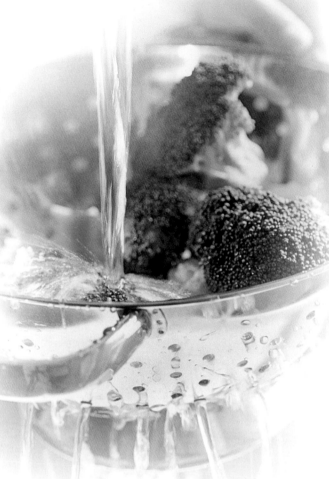

The folate, vitamin C, and calcium in this member of the brassica or cruciferous vegetable family make it a pregnancy essential. Purple-sprouting varieties—staples of farmers' markets and farm shops—have a delicate texture and fine flavor, while larger-headed calabrese are more widely available, being easier to transport. Those who grow their own adore the purple-sprouting type; it fills the traditional gap in the vegetable season and can be harvested for several weeks.

GOOD FOR YOU AND YOUR BABY

Broccoli has the most nutrients of any vegetable. It is an excellent source of folate and vitamins C, K, and beta-carotene. Additionally, it contains manganese, potassium, vitamins B_2 and B_6, phosphorus, magnesium, iron, and calcium, plus omega-3 fatty acids. It is rich in fiber and contains protein. The combination of calcium and vitamin C is bone protecting and boosts the immune system. The phytonutrients found in broccoli, including sulforaphane and indoles, boost detoxification enzymes that protect the cells. The brassica also benefits the cardiovascular system, eyes, and liver and promotes immunity. Japanese studies suggest that compounds in broccoli combat the bacterium H. pylori, a common trigger of gastritis. At John Hopkins University, extracts were used to heal sun-damaged skin.

BUYING NOTES

Choose the most compact and darkest blue- or purple-green heads, which are signs of freshness: fresh broccoli is some 5 percent protein. The stems should be hard and dense, not floppy or light. A hole up the center of the stem is a sign of age. Avoid yellowing florets; beta-carotene clusters in the florets and a lack of color signals a lack of the nutrient. Frozen broccoli florets are a good source of beta-carotene.

GROWING AND HARVESTING NOTES

Because it overwinters, broccoli ties up space in the garden for a whole year, so you might not want to grow it if you only have one bed. Sow in mid-spring to harvest from late winter to spring. Broccoli needs plenty of moisture, and does well in humid climates and in clay soil. Net in early spring against hungry birds.

To harvest, pick before the flower buds open, the clusters separate, or the buds start to yellow, and do so frequently to encourage the plant to send out more shoots. Cut the main head first, then the side florets.

CULINARY DOS AND DON'TS

- Slice into florets and leave for 5 minutes before cooking to promote the availability of phytonutrients.
- Cook quickly (steam, sauté, or stir-fry); phytonutrients are lost when broccoli is cooked for longer than five minutes. Steam to preserve folate and antioxidants and sauté or stir-fry in extra-virgin olive oil. In tests, this was the only oil that maintained the phytonutrient and vitamin C count of raw broccoli.
- Cook the slender flowering shoots upright, as for asparagus, or eat raw.
- If available, use the leaves as you would cabbage; they are a storehouse of nutrients.
- Don't microwave broccoli; in one study this reduced antioxidants by up to 97 percent.

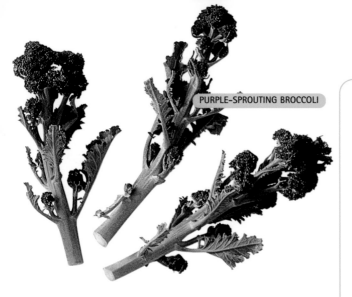

Purple-sprouting broccoli, with its many small clusters of buds and sprue-like stalk, tastes especially good. In 18th-century England it was known as Italian Asparagus. Though the purple variety looks pretty in raw dishes, its color fades in the pan. The tender leaves, stalks, and heads are all edible.

QUICK AND EASY DISHES

- *Serve raw florets as crudités with dips.*
- *Toss blanched florets into salads with chopped sun-dried tomatoes and toasted sunflower seeds.*
- *Drizzle steamed florets with a sesame-seed dressing.*
- *Peel, julienne, and steam or griddle the delicious stems. Serve as for asparagus.*
- *Top cooked broccoli with some grated sharp hard cheese such as cheddar or Parmesan.*
- *Blanch the florets and diced stem, then fry in olive oil with garlic; stir in anchovies and toasted bread crumbs to serve.*
- *Dice a large floret and steam or boil with pasta for an avocado-like sauce.*

CABBAGE, KALE, AND BRUSSELS SPROUTS

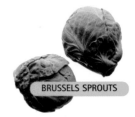

Folklore has it that babies come from the cabbage patch—perhaps because the brassica or cruciferous vegetable family contains so many baby-nurturing nutrients.

Cabbage has been regarded as a cure-all since Classical times; in pregnancy it is useful in reducing morning sickness and afterwards in easing swollen breasts. The robust nature of kale suits hearty stews and winter vegetable soups, while cabbage is a mainstay of Indian dishes; its flavor marries well with spices such as cumin and ginger. All provide vital nutrients, including

----

Add Savoy cabbage to your diet to counter cystitis, and after your milk comes in tuck a Savoy leaf into your bra to relieve painfully swollen breasts. Replace with a new leaf once it has become limp.

----

folate, during the traditional lean months.

The cabbage family is beautifully ornamental in a winter garden, from the deep green crinkly leaves of the Savoy to the glossy heads of red cabbage and Brussels sprouts popping rose-like from their tall stems.

GOOD FOR YOU AND YOUR BABY

Cabbage, kale, and Brussels sprouts are all amazingly rich in vitamins K and C, and contain manganese, B vitamins, folate, calcium, and potassium. Cabbages contain omega-3 fatty acids, as well as fiber and protein. The phytonutrients in cabbage, including sulforaphane and indoles, boost detoxification enzymes that protect the cells. The family also benefits cardiovascular, eye, and liver health and promotes immunity. Red cabbage is rich in anthocyanins (which produce the color) and has particularly high levels of vitamin C, though kale has the most antioxidants of any leafy green. The distinctive taste of Brussels sprouts is a result of the phytonutrient sinigrin, which some people find very bitter.

Cabbage is beneficial for gastrointestinal problems, and a 1989 study found it useful in reducing morning sickness. It seems particularly effective when fermented as sauerkraut (pickled cabbage): this preserves all its vitamin C while adding gastro-friendly bacteria.

BUYING NOTES

Favor cabbages with firm heads and dark leaves. The darker the shade (green or red), the greater the vitamins. Don't throw away the outer leaves, which are especially nutrient-rich, and avoid ready-cut heads—once cut, a cabbage starts to lose vitamin C. Reject anything with yellowing leaves and a squashy texture.

Choose firm, compact Brussels sprouts. Those sold on the stem stay fresh longer than loose ones. The smaller,

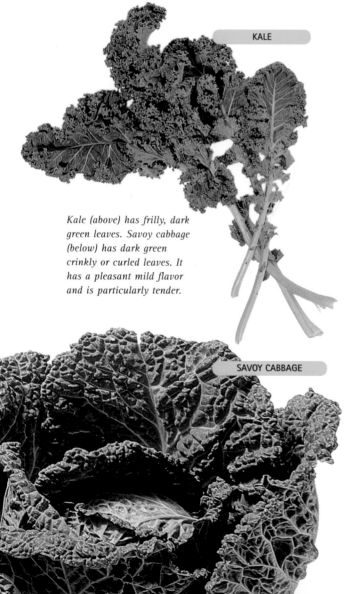

KALE

SAVOY CABBAGE

Kale (above) has frilly, dark green leaves. Savoy cabbage (below) has dark green crinkly or curled leaves. It has a pleasant mild flavor and is particularly tender.

QUICK AND EASY DISHES

- *Sir-fry shredded kale with walnut oil, garlic, and soy sauce.*
- *Sauté shredded kale with garlic and cannellini beans and serve on bruschetta with Parmesan.*
- *Use shredded cabbage as a base for salad, with walnuts, apple, and celery.*
- *Throw bok choy into stir-fries and Chinese soups.*
- *Mix shredded cabbage with mashed potato and finely chopped onion; fry in a little olive oil until it has a crispy crust and serve with cold meat.*
- *Braise red cabbage in orange juice with a little balsamic vinegar, honey, and star anise over low heat for around two hours to accompany red meat and game.*
- *Try Brussels spouts raw: shred and serve with a vinaigrette, or blanch, then pan-fry with a little butter and bacon.*
- *Lightly steam Brussels sprouts or kale then sauté with cooked chestnuts and bacon or lardons.*

greener ones have the sweetest taste. If buying kale, choose small bunches with crispy leaves. Go organic to avoid high levels of pesticides. In 2009 the Environmental Working Group in the US identified it as one of the 12 most pesticide-contaminated foods.

GROWING AND HARVESTING NOTES

If you plan ingeniously, you can cut fresh cabbages year-round. This family does well by the sea, which gives a clue to their favored climate—a cool humidity characterized by mizzle (mist and a moist soil). Perfect for pregnancy gardening, cabbages don't need much attention and require firm soil, so you don't have to do lots of digging. But do net seedlings to deter flying pests and birds, and maintain a slug and snail watch during the early weeks. Later in the season, make sure that caterpillars and their eggs are picked off.

Cabbages divide into seasonal groups: spring, summer, autumn, and hardy winter, so plan successional sowings. Curly kale is extremely hardy and tends to thrive for even the laziest gardener. Remove yellowing leaves to prevent rotting and aid air circulation. Cut the kale leaves young (avoiding the lower leaves) and leave the plants in situ to resprout and grow into heads.

CULINARY DOS AND DON'TS

- Eat cabbage raw, lightly steamed, or stir-fried for maximum nutrients.
- Slice or shred and leave for five minutes before cooking to promote the availability of phytonutrients.
- Stir-fry finely chopped leaves in a little olive oil to maximize nutrient uptake.
- If adding cabbage leaves to stews and soups, do so a few minutes before serving rather than leaving them to cook for a lengthy period.
- Discard kale stems before cooking. The first shoots are less pungent than full-grown leaves with a softer texture; they can be added to salads or stir-fries.
- Wash greens in cold water, pat dry and store in a plastic bag lined with paper towels in the refrigerator for up to three days.

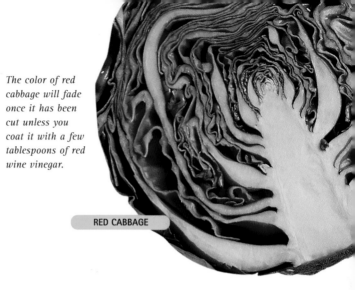

The color of red cabbage will fade once it has been cut unless you coat it with a few tablespoons of red wine vinegar.

RED CABBAGE

SPINACH AND SWISS CHARD

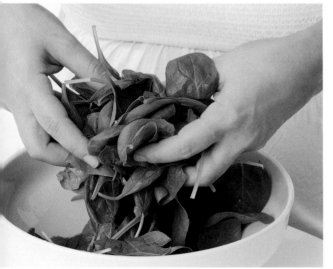

These leafy greens pack a punch in terms of flavor and pregnancy nutrients. Spinach is best known as a tonic for pregnancy anemia. An old wives' tale is that it makes baby's hair curl! The plants are incredibly easy to raise at home, which is useful when so many nutrients are lost in transit and storage. Both make perfect cut-and-come-again plants (see page 40).

Chard resembles spinach in flavor, but is a form of beet bred for its leaves. The stunning purple-red, rose, or yellow stems of the ruby variety are ornamental as well as tasty. Both chard and spinach hold their own in robust-flavor combinations, and are often used in Middle Eastern and Indian recipes.

GOOD FOR YOU AND YOUR BABY

Spinach contains more protein than any other leafy vegetable and is an excellent source of vitamin K and beta-carotene, folate, manganese, magnesium, and iron. It contains good amounts of vitamins C, B_2, B_6 and E, calcium, potassium, copper, and zinc. It's great for fiber, too. Spinach contains at least 13 antioxidants, including flavonoids, and together the vitamin K, calcium, and magnesium build bones. The copper promotes uptake of the iron in red blood cells. Spinach is helpful in lowering blood pressure and promoting gastrointestinal health. It also has anti-inflammatory properties.

Cooked spinach is best for iron content but contains oxalic acid, which restricts calcium and iron absorption. Swiss chard has similar properties to spinach, but less oxalic acid. It is therefore recommended to wait for a few hours before eating other iron- and calcium-rich foods or to eat these oxalate-rich foods with a source of vitamin C (such as orange juice) to boost iron uptake.

BUYING NOTES

The darker the leaves, the greater the nutrients. Look for firm stalks and crisp and unblemished leaves; avoid discolored and limp leaves and stems. It is better to choose frozen than week-old leaves.

PLANTING UP A CONTAINER

The principle is the same, whether planting up long, narrow window boxes or deep half-barrels. Before you begin, check that the container is large enough and deep enough for the plants you plan to raise, and make sure it has drainage holes. You will need someone to help you lift large bags of potting compost and maneuver containers into place.

Make sure the container is in its final position and have the plants or seeds ready nearby.

1 Raise pots off the ground with specially made terra-cotta "feet," wooden blocks, or bricks; place a drip tray underneath window boxes. Place a layer of "crocks" (terra-cotta pieces) or gravel at the bottom of the container, to aid drainage.

2 Add peat-free, multipurpose compost (or soil suitable for your plants) over the gravel or crocks. Fill to within 1 inch of the top of the container, flattening down the compost with your hands to remove air pockets. Water well.

3 Transplant young plants or sow seeds (follow the packet directions). If using plants, loosen the roots before adding to the container.

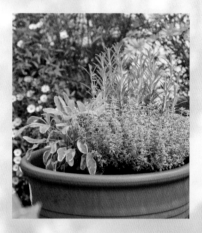

4 Sit all plants at the same level in the pot and firm the compost around them. Water carefully so as not to uproot the plants (or disturb the seeds).

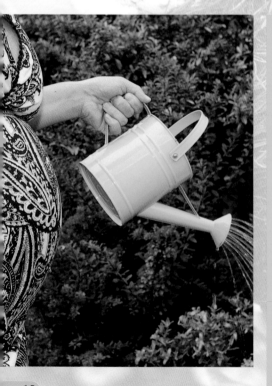

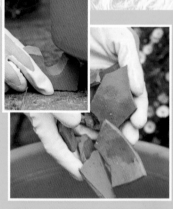

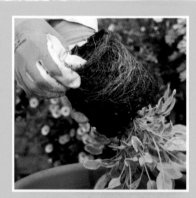

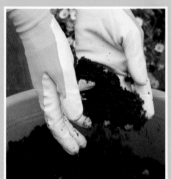

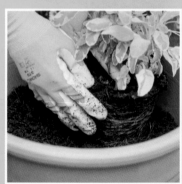

PLANTING UP A HANGING BASKET

Choose the deepest, widest basket you can find to cut down on watering—more soil means less moisture loss—and search out a lightweight potting compost. Before you begin, mix the compost with some water retention granules to, again, cut down on watering. "Tumbler" cherry tomatoes and dwarfing peas and beans look attractive trailing over the sides of the basket.

1 Stand the basket on a pot or bucket to keep it stable. Line the basket with fiber lining from a garden center and heavy-duty plastic to retain moisture. Make some drainage slits in the bottom and sides of the lining.

2 Fill the basket half-full with potting compost and add up to 3 plants, depending on basket size.

3 Top up the compost to within 1 inch of the top of the basket. Firm around the plants.

4 Water well before asking someone to hang the basket (at a height you can reach). Feed weekly when the crops begin to set.

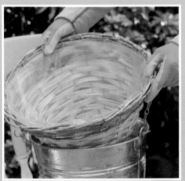

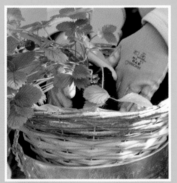

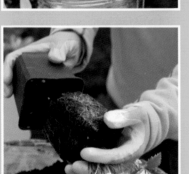

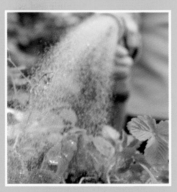

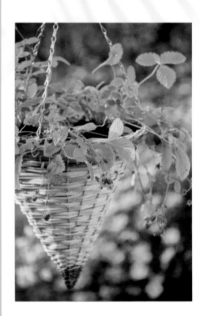

GROWING AND HARVESTING NOTES

Spinach and chard are incredibly easy to grow—some gardeners even consider them weeds because they self-sow if left to run to seed. As well as being low maintenance, they tolerate poor soil. You need never be without spinach if you plant summer and winter varieties; make several sowings for successional harvesting, but be vigilant during warmer weather, when plants have a tendency to bolt.

You can happily neglect Swiss chard as the leaves are rarely attacked by slugs. Plant in a planter or at the front of a border for show as well as easy picking. Chard is grown chiefly for the stalk; pull stalks when harvesting rather than cutting.

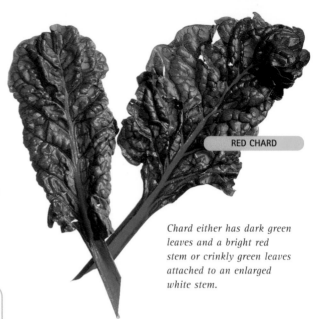

RED CHARD

Chard either has dark green leaves and a bright red stem or crinkly green leaves attached to an enlarged white stem.

FOLATE-BOOST TONIC

This juice is a general tonic when you feel in need of pepping up. The spinach may ease constipation and strengthen bleeding gums; it is also valued for its skin-regenerating properties. Try to buy organic produce. You will need a juicer.

> 4½ cups spinach
> 1 stick celery
> 1 carrot
> ¾ cup tomato juice
> Worcestershire sauce (optional)

Wash the spinach leaves well and remove any thick stems. Place the leaves in a pan, cover and cook over medium heat for 2–3 minutes. Put the carrot and celery through the juicer, then the cooked spinach. Pour into a pitcher and stir in the tomato juice. Pour into a glass over ice and serve with a few shakes of Worcestershire sauce, if using. Store any remaining juice in the refrigerator for up to 24 hours.

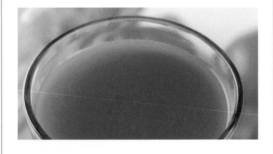

QUICK AND EASY DISHES
* *Spinach is very good with eggs; steam the leaves, then chop and stir in a little grated nutmeg and Parmesan, and top with poached eggs.*

CULINARY DOS AND DON'TS
* Young leaves are most palatable. Discard the ribs of older spinach leaves before cooking.
* Eat spinach raw (after washing well) for maximum nutrient absorption.
* Combine spinach with a source of vitamin C, such as sliced red bell pepper, to boost mineral absorption.
* Drizzle spinach leaves with olive or walnut oil to promote the uptake of vitamin E and the phytonutrient lutein, which protects the eyes.
* Cook more spinach than you think you need to allow for shrinkage during cooking—about 4½ cups per person.
* Don't add water when cooking spinach, just rinse the leaves, place in a pan over low heat and cover. Allow to sweat for a few minutes until the leaves have melted into a soft mound. Squeeze out the remaining moisture, chop and serve.
* The longer you store spinach, the less folate and fewer carotenoids. Chard keeps better than spinach.
* Cut off the leaves and simmer chard stems; serve as for asparagus.

⚘ BEETS

Another fabulous, folate-rich food, beet comes into its own at lunchtime if you are prone to afternoon energy dips, because it converts to sugar extremely slowly and keeps blood-sugar levels stable. The root has long been used medicinally to support the blood and digestion and as a natural laxative. One of the best reasons for growing beet yourself is to have a ready supply of young leaves: they are from the same family as spinach and Swiss chard. You won't find the leaves in supermarkets; indeed, they wilt so quickly they're rarely found at farmers' markets.

GOOD FOR YOU AND YOUR BABY
As well as supplying excellent amounts of folate, beets contain very good levels of manganese and potassium and are a good source of vitamin C, magnesium, phosphorus, copper, and iron. The copper promotes the uptake of the iron in red blood cells. The leaves are a great source of iron and calcium—they have more than spinach—and are also very high in beta-carotene and vitamin C.

The red color highlights the plant's beneficial properties. The antioxidant betalain pigments, betacyanin (purple) and betaxanthin (yellow), support the liver and boost immune function. Antioxidant carotenoids and flavonoids also boost immunity and cardiovascular health and reduce inflammation. Beet seems to be able to neutralize dangerous nitrates if you've been eating processed meats.

A study by Barts and the London School of Medicine and the Peninsula Medical School found that drinking 2 cups of beet juice daily reduced blood pressure. University of Exeter research suggests that drinking the

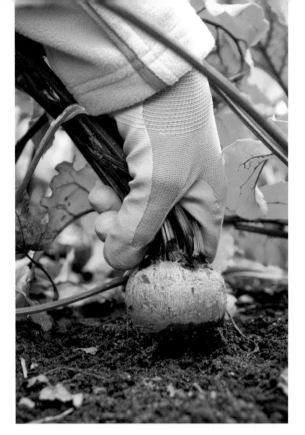

If growing your own, you can store any leftover roots in a cool, dark place. The traditional method is to store the roots in layers in a box covered in sand.

juice increases stamina, helping to make strenuous activity less tiring (you might like to sip it in the early stages of labor).

Beets, especially the leaves, contain oxalic acid, which can prevent calcium and iron absorption. It is therefore recommended to wait for a few hours before eating iron and calcium-rich foods or to eat beets with a source of vitamin C (orange juice) to boost iron uptake. It will color your urine and stools pink, but that's completely harmless.

BUYING NOTES
Small- and medium-size beets are juicier than larger ones. Look for bunches with leaves—a clue to how old the roots are. The leaves should be fresh and springy to the touch. The root should be firm, unwrinkled, and with no soft patches. Press the root before buying—lots of give means the vegetable is past its best. Avoid ready-cooked, vacuum-packed beet, which tends to taste of nothing or of vinegar.

QUICK AND EASY DISHES
- *Add raw, shredded beets to salads or stir into plain yogurt.*
- *Dress young leaves with olive oil, vinegar, and seasoning.*
- *Roasting the root brings out its sweetness; chop and add to the roasting pan alongside other winter staples, such as carrots, parsnips, celeriac, and squash.*

GROWING AND HARVESTING NOTES

Sow in succession to ensure a crop from late spring to fall. If at first the young plants seem to stall, let them be—they take a while to get going. Once they have, thin seedlings so they do not touch; this encourages the root to swell. You can leave the roots in situ into mild winters, though watch that they don't get too tough, or store in a sand-covered box.

Twist off the leaves rather than cutting to prevent the root from bleeding.

CULINARY DOS AND DON'TS

- Eat the leaves raw (after washing well) for maximum absorption of minerals.
- The root can be shredded and used in salads.
- Combine the root with a source of vitamin C, such as broccoli, sweet peppers, and lemon juice to boost mineral absorption.
- Cooking increases the availability of beta-carotene and fiber but steam, microwave, or roast to preserve the levels of vitamin C and B.
- Don't overdo the vinegar; this can drown the earthy subtlety of flavor.
- Don't boil the root; this will destroy vital nutrients.

PURPLE ENERGY JUICE

The nitrate in the beet has been shown to boost stamina, keeping you going when energy is flagging. Beet is also soothing for pregnancy constipation. The ginger in the juice helps to combat nausea. You will need a juicer.

1 medium raw beet (organic, if possible)
1 inch fresh ginger root
1 apple

Top and tail, then peel the beet (take care, the juice stains); peel the ginger and wash the apple. Put all the ingredients through the juicer. Store any leftover juice in the refrigerator for up to 48 hours.

PEAS AND SNOW PEAS

Excellent for healthy bones and a good source of folate, peas can be a tonic for the soul. What could be more uplifting than popping the juicy contents from a fresh pod straight into your mouth? Supermarket peas often lack the flavor and sweetness of home-grown ones or those found in farmers' markets. Pea pods are a perfect portable snack during pregnancy, as are mangetout, the young pods eaten whole. Sugar snaps have a crunchier texture and are sweeter than garden peas.

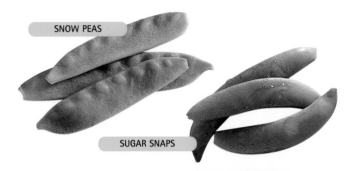

SNOW PEAS

SUGAR SNAPS

GOOD FOR YOU AND YOUR BABY

A very good source of vitamins B_1, C and K, manganese, and folate, peas contain good amounts, too, of vitamins A and B_6, phosphorus, magnesium, copper, iron, and zinc. The copper promotes the uptake of iron in red blood cells. Peas are great for fiber and protein and also contain antioxidant betalain and carotenoids, which support the cardiovascular and immune systems.

BUYING NOTES

Look for firm, bright green pods; be wary of those that shake—the peas inside won't be fully grown. Frozen peas may be fresher, tastier and more nutritious than podded peas past their best. When selecting snow or sugar snap peas, choose smaller pods, avoiding those that are ready topped and tailed.

Eat the peas the day you buy the pods; they are tastiest when just picked.

GROWING AND HARVESTING NOTES

Peas like manured, well-dug soil with good drainage, so get someone to do this for you. Successional planting is essential to prevent gluts: sow every 2–3 weeks from mid-spring, or even earlier for a chance crop. Net young plants and mulch around them to cut back on weeding (they like it cool and damp). After picking, cut back the plants, but leave the roots in the ground to shed nitrogen into the soil. Follow on with a nitrogen-loving crop such as cabbage, spinach, or lettuce. Don't plant peas in the same bed two years running.

To cut down on work, choose self-supporting varieties, which require less staking and make easier picking (no grubbing around under collapsed pea sticks). You can pick young shelling peas to eat as snow peas, or grow specific snow pea varieties.

Pick regularly to encourage the plant to make more flowers. Pick snow peas when the pod is still flat, but the first bumps of young peas are pushing through.

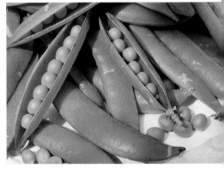

They should snap crisply, or allow to mature and pick to shell. Once pods fade from bright green, the peas will be tough. To harvest dried peas, leave on the plant; once the pods have dried to a husk, cut off the whole plant and hang until completely dry. Pod the dried peas and store in an airtight jar in a cool, dark place ready to be rehydrated by soaking.

CULINARY DOS AND DON'TS

- Eat freshly picked peas raw for the sweetest taste.
- Cook fresh peas only 2–3 minutes in boiling water. Throw a few empty pods into the cooking water for extra flavor.
- It's traditional to cook peas between layers of firm-leafed lettuce; add a couple of tablespoons of water for steaming.
- Add uncooked snow peas to salads.
- If cooking snow peas, steam or stir-fry.

QUICK AND EASY DISHES

- *Serve peas with a little butter and a few torn leaves of fresh mint.*
- *Add a handful of peas to cooked rice or risotto or combine with pasta.*

peas and snow peas

FAVA BEANS

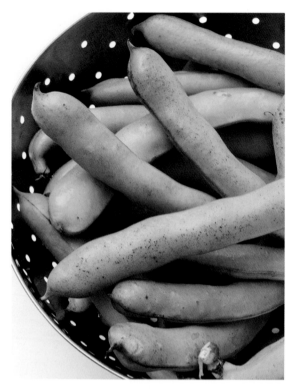

Young and fresh fava beans, also known as broad beans, have a pleasant texture and sweet taste.

fava beans retain their flavor remarkably well, and are a better choice than older, fresh pods.

GROWING AND HARVESTING NOTES
Easy to grow, fava beans need little tending, tolerate most soils, and do well in dry conditions. Sow a batch mid-late fall, well mulched, to overwinter for a late spring crop that contributes attractive black and white ornamental flowers. Sow another batch in early spring to chase them. After harvesting, leave the roots in the ground to shed their nitrogen. Follow with a nitrogen-loving crop such as lettuce, cabbage, or spinach. Don't grow beans in the same bed two years running. To deter black fly, pinch out the flowering tops.

Longpod types contain more beans (eight) and are hardier, while Windsor cultivars have fewer beans (four or five), but are considered finer in flavor. Fava beans are usually green, but look for bronze or pink heirloom varieties. Choose varieties that need no staking to cut down on work.

You can harvest the beans young (to eat like snow peas), as mature pods, or leave until they have shriveled on the plant to store dried. Pick the pods regularly to encourage the plant to make more flowers. Fava beans are wonderfully tactile to pod with their cotton-wool soft interior.

CULINARY DOS AND DON'TS
- Simply top and tail very young pods and eat raw or cook whole, as you would snow peas.
- Use the young leafy tops like collard greens.
- Eat fava beans as soon as possible for the sweetest flavor and softest texture.
- For older beans, slide off the outer skin before cooking for the best flavor.

Before the arrival of the potato, fava beans were a staple food in Europe, which says a great deal about their nutrient profile. Since antiquity, they have been associated with magical growth, abundance, new life, and rebirth—perhaps because they arrive early in the growing season and, once dried, nourish through the winter. Like corn, this is an ingredient whose flavor benefits from as short a journey from plant to pot as possible, making them ideal for the garden.

GOOD FOR YOU AND YOUR BABY
Fava beans are a very good source of folate, and also contain phosphorus, manganese, magnesium, potassium, iron, and copper; the last promotes the uptake of iron in red blood cells. They also contain B vitamins and are full of fiber and protein. Since they contain the "feel-good" chemical L-dopa, fava beans may perk you up when you feel worried or despondent.

BUYING NOTES
Avoid pods that look withered or are soft. Beans that have been on display too long will be tough; frozen

> ### QUICK AND EASY DISHES
> - *Add a little parsley to cooked fava beans.*
> - *For a snack, try habas fritas (roasted Spanish fava beans).*

GREEN AND RUNNER BEANS

Green beans, also known as French or string beans, have three incarnations. The whole pod can be eaten fresh while young; when mature, the beans can be eaten green (known as flageolets); or they can be dried, when they are known as white beans. These beans come in many varieties, shapes, and colors, and have longevity at the end of the harvest season. Flageolets make especially fine eating.

GOOD FOR YOU AND YOUR BABY

Beans contain vitamins C, A and K and manganese aplenty, and are a good source of folate. They also contain potassium, magnesium, vitamins B_1 and B_2, iron, and copper, which promotes the uptake of iron in red blood cells. Importantly, beans contain omega-3 fatty acids and are packed with fiber and protein.

Be aware that dried beans contain the starches stachyose and raffinose, which are indigestible and can cause discomfort and wind.

BUYING NOTES

When buying fresh, choose bright green, smooth beans. Break one to test for freshness—fresh ones will snap; older ones bend and have stringy sides. Avoid beans with spots. Good runner beans are tricky to find fresh in supermarkets, which may be why so many people choose to grow their own. Source dried green flageolets from gourmet storesor heirloom websites if they're not in your local supermarket. The original French variety, Chevrier Vert, has the best flavor. Frozen beans contain more vitamin C than week-old fresh produce.

GROWING AND HARVESTING NOTES

Green and runner beans suit lazy winter gardeners; they can't be sown until late in the season, after all chance of frost is finished. The seeds need plenty of food and moisture: get someone to dig a deep trench early in the year and throw in your kitchen compost, waiting until late spring to sow—any earlier and the cold may prevent germination. It's often as effective to sow directly outdoors, another labor-saving method. Train climbing beans up canes tied into tripods or A-frames connected with an extra cane for a colorful display and easy picking. After harvesting, leave the roots in the ground to shed their nitrogen. Follow on with a nitrogen-loving crop such as spinach or lettuce. Never grow beans in the same bed two years running. Keep a vigilant slug watch while plants are young.

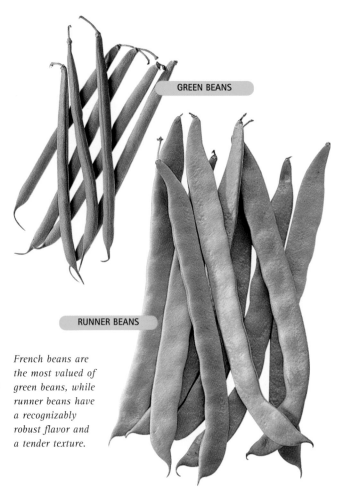

GREEN BEANS

RUNNER BEANS

French beans are the most valued of green beans, while runner beans have a recognizably robust flavor and a tender texture.

The pods of green beans may be round or flat, thin or wide, and range in color from bluish-purple to white splattered with yellow (they shed the purple in the pan). Few interesting varieties are found in supermarkets, which is why they are fun to grow. Buy non-hybrid seed so you can dry beans to sow next year. Sow vigorous climbing beans for a long show and plenty of pods, or dwarfing bush cultivars for a quicker crop and less staking but a shorter harvest.

Scarlet-bloomed runner beans are showiest of all for the summer garden, very vigorous and incredibly tasty, but all beans are nutritious and filling.

Beans are perfect for picking during pregnancy, since you don't have to bend over. Pick regularly to encourage the plant to make more flowers. Eat whole green beans young, before the bean inside has matured.

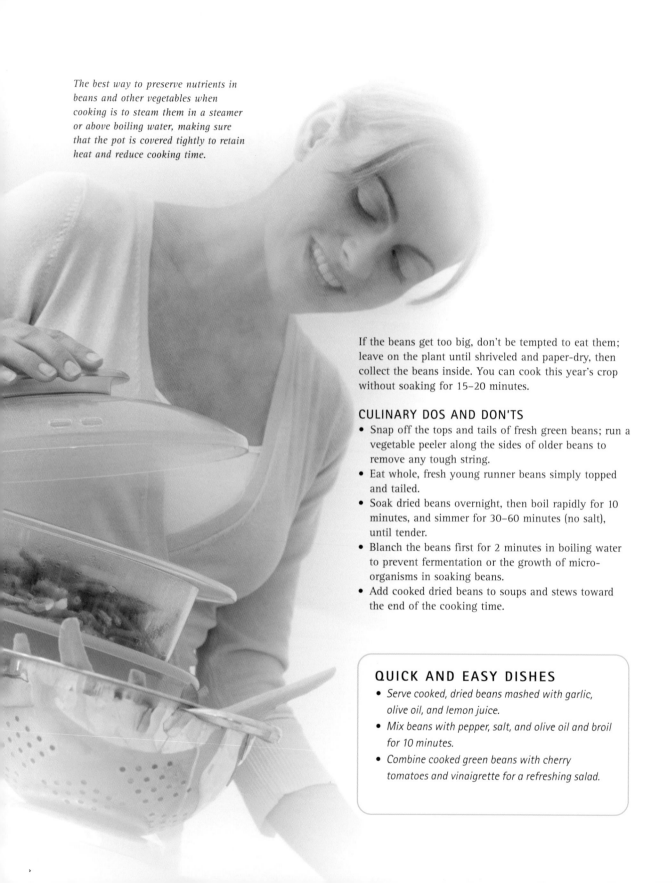

The best way to preserve nutrients in beans and other vegetables when cooking is to steam them in a steamer or above boiling water, making sure that the pot is covered tightly to retain heat and reduce cooking time.

If the beans get too big, don't be tempted to eat them; leave on the plant until shriveled and paper-dry, then collect the beans inside. You can cook this year's crop without soaking for 15–20 minutes.

CULINARY DOS AND DON'TS

- Snap off the tops and tails of fresh green beans; run a vegetable peeler along the sides of older beans to remove any tough string.
- Eat whole, fresh young runner beans simply topped and tailed.
- Soak dried beans overnight, then boil rapidly for 10 minutes, and simmer for 30–60 minutes (no salt), until tender.
- Blanch the beans first for 2 minutes in boiling water to prevent fermentation or the growth of micro-organisms in soaking beans.
- Add cooked dried beans to soups and stews toward the end of the cooking time.

QUICK AND EASY DISHES

- *Serve cooked, dried beans mashed with garlic, olive oil, and lemon juice.*
- *Mix beans with pepper, salt, and olive oil and broil for 10 minutes.*
- *Combine cooked green beans with cherry tomatoes and vinaigrette for a refreshing salad.*

ASPARAGUS

Among the most folate-filled vegetables, asparagus spears are a treat in the first trimester. They never taste better than when bought from a local grower or picked at home. Those that have traveled the globe tend to be light in taste. Starting an asparagus bed is like having a baby—a long-term project not to be undertaken lightly. It will usually be two to three years before you are over the teething troubles and into pleasure. But an asparagus bed should still be productive when your child has left home—think of it as a living heirloom.

GOOD FOR YOU AND YOUR BABY

Packed with folate and vitamin K, plus vitamin C and beta-carotene, B vitamins, manganese, potassium, copper, and iron, asparagus also contains protein and fiber. The spears contain inulin, which supports friendly bacteria in the gut.

Asparagus has a diuretic effect; it has been used since ancient times as a cure for swelling and water retention,

----

Don't worry if your urine smells after eating asparagus; it's the constituent amino acid methionine, which is harmless.

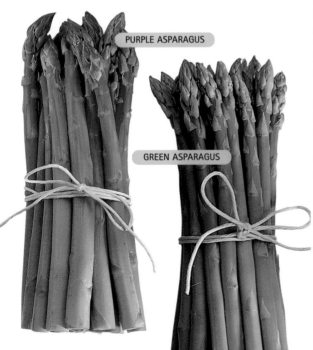

PURPLE ASPARAGUS

GREEN ASPARAGUS

QUICK AND EASY DISHES

- *Broil spears with a drizzle of olive oil, turning to char-broil evenly; add a squeeze of lemon juice and black pepper to serve.*
- *Serve simply, with melted butter or a lemony vinaigrette.*
- *Shave Parmesan over grilled spears.*
- *Try serving asparagus with eggs; a delicious combination.*
- *Toss chopped, cooked spears in a creamy pasta sauce.*

and can ease cystitis. In Ayurvedic medicine, asparagus is used to boost female fertility.

BUYING NOTES

Choose locally grown vegetables over those that have traveled. This means eating in season, from mid-spring to early summer. At farmers' markets you may come across cheaper "kitchen-grade" spears, which make perfect eating, but are too thin or short for the supermarket. They are a bargain. Thin spears (or "sprue") are tastier than giant stalks that stand up well to freighting. If you happen to grow your own, asparagus numbers among the crops that taste best when picked while the cooking water is rising to a boil. Canned or bottled asparagus will help you maintain healthy digestive flora, but is flavor-free.

Creating an asparagus bed is a major undertaking since you need to give over enough space for 30 crowns, then leave it in place for 20 years. Most crowns cannot be cropped in the first two or three years.

CULINARY DOS AND DON'TS

- Choose green or purple spears over white as they have more phytonutrients.
- Cut off the woody ends.
- Don't peel the spears; just rinse well.
- If you don't have an asparagus kettle, tie in a loose bundle and cook upright in a large pot, covering with foil to steam the tips.
- Asparagus spears are ready after about 5 minutes, depending on thickness, but a little bite is good.

❧ WINTER SQUASH

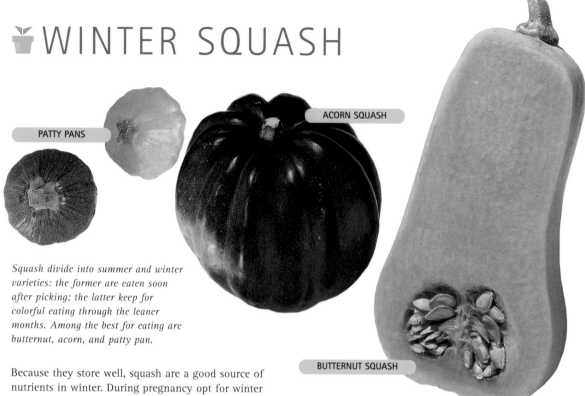

PATTY PANS

ACORN SQUASH

BUTTERNUT SQUASH

Squash divide into summer and winter varieties: the former are eaten soon after picking; the latter keep for colorful eating through the leaner months. Among the best for eating are butternut, acorn, and patty pan.

Because they store well, squash are a good source of nutrients in winter. During pregnancy opt for winter varieties over summer's zucchini; they are tastier and contain more nutrients. Squash and pumpkins are symbols of motherly abundance in some cultures: in the Congo, a young woman may be massaged with white squash to make her as fertile as the plant itself! As a basic rule, the deeper colored the flesh, the more phytonutrients (and taste).

GOOD FOR YOU AND YOUR BABY
Winter squash are high in beta-carotene, unlike the summer variety, and are also a very good source of vitamin C, potassium, and manganese, as well as containing good amounts of folate, B vitamins, omega-3 fatty acids, and copper. They are fiber-filled and contain high levels of the orange-red carotenoid beta-cryptoxanthin, which supports lung health, as well as antioxidant and anti-inflammatory beta-carotene. The seeds are a ready source of omega-3 fatty acids and zinc, vitamin E, magnesium, and folate, and have the ability to lower levels of cholesterol.

BUYING NOTES
Avoid huge pumpkins raised for Halloween (for easy-cut flesh). Select for heaviness and firmness instead. You'll find more unusual varieties at the farmers' market or at farm shops. Don't touch those that have blemishes or soft patches.

GROWING AND HARVESTING NOTES
These plants like lots of food, so get someone to work in lots of manure or compost before planting out. Don't transplant young plants until all danger of frost has passed, and then maintain a slug watch. Try inverting glass jars over young plants at the end of the day, as if tucking them into bed. As they grow, the plants require plenty of water as well as lots of room to sprawl, so mulch well to make your task easier. Water especially attentively when the flowers are forming and fruit setting. To make the most of the foliage and flowers (and to tame growth in a smaller space), train the plants up a fence or over a pergola. It's traditional to interplant to grow up through corn and beans. "Stop" plants to

> ## QUICK AND EASY DISHES
> - *Add a pinch each of dried cumin, coriander, and ginger to cooked squash*
> - *Scoop out pumpkin seeds, wash and spread on a baking sheet in a low oven until toasted; serve with a little salt.*

goodness from the garden

28

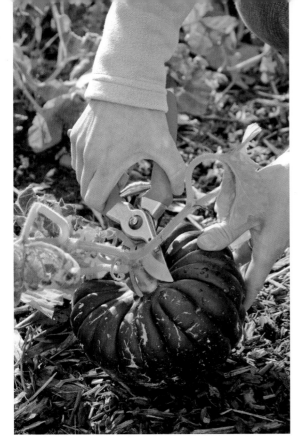

When harvesting squash, cut them from the vine with the stem attached. Check for ripeness by examining color, texture, and firmness.

encourage larger fruit by nipping off extra flowers and fruit so that only two or three can develop per plant. Cut away mildewed leaves and any shading the fruit to allow it to mature.

Leave squash on the vine as long as possible to become dense, even after the leaves have gone. After cutting mature pumpkins and squash (with a long stem for easy carrying), leave them to cure, or harden, in the autumn sun for around two weeks (bring them in if temperatures drop). When ready, they sound hollow when tapped and the skin is tough. Use those with blemishes or bite holes at once; others you can store for two to six months.

CULINARY DOS AND DON'TS

- Turn winter squash into satisfying soups with the addition of a little curry powder if your pregnancy palate will allow; stir in yogurt to cool.
- Use seaweed salt to bring out the buttery flavor.
- Brush slices of pumpkin with honey before roasting.

POTATOES

Many of us gravitate toward comfort food during pregnancy, and few dishes are as comforting as a bowl of fluffy mashed potato. Indeed, potato's botanical name, *Solanum tuberosum*, derives from a Latin term meaning "soothing." Don't stress about bad carbs: potatoes are a good nutrient source.

GOOD FOR YOU AND YOUR BABY

Potatoes supply vitamins C and B_6, and some copper, potassium, and manganese. They contain fiber, too. Potatoes are rich in antioxidant plant compounds that protect against heart disease and respiratory problems and lower blood pressure. The starch in cold boiled potatoes supports healthy digestive flora. Potatoes can raise blood-sugar levels quickly; calm yourself by teaming them with peas, beans, or yogurt. Tradition holds that a potato in the pocket cures pregnancy piles!

Sweet potatoes, which are unrelated to the common potato, are much higher in antioxidant phytonutrients,

beta-carotene, manganese, and vitamins C and B_6. They also contain copper, potassium, and iron. In all potatoes, nutrients are concentrated in and just below the skin.

BUYING NOTES

The longer potatoes are stored, the fewer nutrients they have—blemishes and softness are a sign of age. Avoid ready-scrubbed potatoes in plastic bags; plastic makes them produce sweat and rot. Those covered in soil will keep longer. Throw away sprouted potatoes and any with a hint of green; they contain the alkaloid solanine, a poison. Choose waxy, yellow-fleshed potatoes to boil, steam or sauté and to use in salads. Choose starchy varieties for baking, mashing, and roasting.

When choosing sweet potatoes, the darker the color, the better the flavor and moistness and the more antioxidants. There are two types: one has orange-red skin and deep pink flesh, the other has a darker, almost purplish skin and paler flesh.

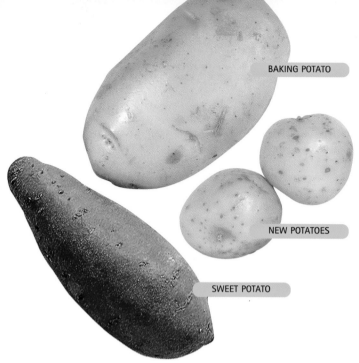

BAKING POTATO

NEW POTATOES

SWEET POTATO

CULINARY DOS AND DON'TS

- Eat new potatoes quickly; they don't keep.
- Cook organic potatoes in the skin to preserve nutrients.
- Don't peel new potatoes; the skins haven't fully matured and contribute flavor.
- Parboil potatoes for 3 minutes before roasting, drain well and toss smartly in the pan. This textures the outside for extra crispiness.
- Sprinkle roast potatoes with chunky sea salt before roasting.
- For perfect baked potatoes, prick the outsides all over with a fork and rub in olive oil and sea salt.
- Bake or roast sweet potatoes—they need less time than regular potatoes. When baking, wrapping in foil preserves nutrients.
- Store potatoes in a cool, dark place, preferably in a burlap sack.

GROWING AND HARVESTING NOTES

Potatoes are perfect for new gardens, reputed to "clean" and break up compacted soil, but do best if plenty of compost is worked into the soil the fall before planting (ask someone to do this for you). They grow from seed potato tubers. Look for local varieties and buy as soon as they appear on the shelves. The tubers need to be "chitted": leave in egg boxes in a light, cool room with the eyes facing upward until shoots grow (about six weeks). First earlies give a crop in early summer, when particularly welcome. They are best for taste and require less space than big-cropping mains. Choose earlies if you need to free up soil for a follow-on crop. Earlies are fast pursued by second earlies, then main crop, which extend the growing season into fall and produce larger quantities.

For no-fuss gardening, don't dig. Place the potatoes on the soil and cover with compost or grass clippings. Earth up around the stems to stop the potatoes going green. Potatoes are easily grown in large planters (up to 3 feet wide and deep). Add two plants per container.

Sweet potatoes are a different species and require months of warm weather to thrive and crop, but are relatively easy to grow. Start with slips (available by mail-order) and allow them to trail or train up a tripod.

Potatoes are ready when the first white flowers show, but you can leave in main crops until the leaves have died. To preserve the nutrients, leave potatoes in the ground over winter (as long as there is no frost), harvesting as you need them.

QUICK AND EASY DISHES

- *Add a dollop of yogurt and plenty of black pepper to mash. Make mash richer with olive oil and Parmesan cheese.*
- *Try garlic mashed potatoes made with crushed garlic and a fruity olive oil.*
- *Scoop out the insides of baked potatoes and combine with hard-cooked eggs, scallion, and anchovies. Pile back in the skin, top with Parmesan cheese, and broil to brown the tops.*
- *For potato salad, combine just-cooked new potatoes with chives and sour cream.*
- *For a filling lunch dish, slice large potatoes so thinly you can see through them, wash, pat dry, then layer in a heatproof dish with slices of onion, and pour over vegetable or chicken stock. Top with a tasty hard cheese and bake.*
- *Make a pie filling with mashed sweet potato, ripe bananas, and a little cinnamon and maple syrup.*

PARSNIPS

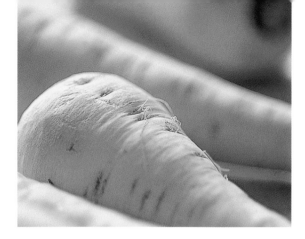

With their earthy sweetness and filling starchiness, parsnips make a useful and nutrient-rich comfort food when it's difficult to stomach ingredients with pronounced flavor or acidity. They are useful in a home vegetable patch because they overwinter in the ground, turning your garden into a convenience store.

GOOD FOR YOU AND YOUR BABY
Parsnips are rich in vitamin C and folate, copper, and manganese. They also contain B vitamins, vitamin K, magnesium, and potassium. They are great for fiber: parsnips contain double the fiber of carrots and more than half is the soluble kind, which can curb blood-sugar swings. The phenolic compounds in parsnips have been associated with relief from dry skin conditions and they support the cardiovascular system.

BUYING NOTES
Smaller and medium-size parsnips are less likely to have a woody or wooly texture; large ones will have a woody center. If you can bend the root, leave it in the store. Ditto those with spots or blemishes. Cut off any green leaves before storing to prevent moisture-loss.

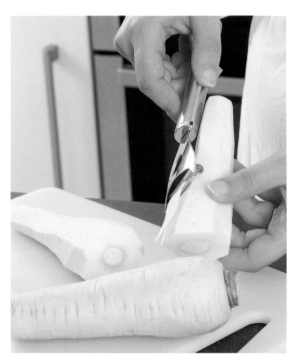

QUICK AND EASY DISHES
- *Drizzle roasted parsnips with a little maple syrup and sprinkle with sesame seeds.*
- *Shred and combine with corn kernels and diced red bell pepper; bind with eggs, form into patties, and fry on each side.*

GROWING AND HARVESTING NOTES
Sow from newly bought seed; some people like to sow into cones of newspaper filled with potting compost. Wait to sow until mid or even late spring for the best chance of success. The long growing season ties up a parsnip bed for much of the year, so plan around them. Interplant with Love-in-a-mist to deter carrot fly; this creates a lovely cottage-garden effect.

On shallow soil choose cultivars with short, fat roots, rather than the traditional types with their long, narrow carrot-like shape.

A dose of frost amplifies the flavor, making parsnips extra sweet, so leave them in the ground over winter, digging up as needed until the spring. Mark the position, so you can find the roots once the foliage dies.

CULINARY DOS AND DON'TS
- You don't have to peel tender young parsnips, just scrub well under running cold water.
- Serve mashed as an alternative to mashed potato; substitute for carrots in stir-fries.
- Add to winter stews left whole or cut in half.
- Halve or quarter parsnips and place in the roasting pan with meat for at least 30 minutes to soak up the flavors.

CARROTS

Carrots are proof that if you enjoy healthy eating during pregnancy, your baby will instinctively follow suit. In one study, the infants of mothers who enjoyed carrot juice lapped it up with their baby cereal; the control group tended to spit it out. In China, eating plenty of carrots in the days before conception is thought to ensure a boy. In Europe, they say it creates a child with red hair and a temper to match!

GOOD FOR YOU AND YOUR BABY

Carrots are the richest vegetable source of beta-carotene and a very good source of vitamins C and K and potassium. They also contain vitamins B_1 and B_6, manganese, some folate, and lots of fiber. Foods rich in carotenoids benefit the skin, eyesight, immune system, and lungs, and can stabilize blood-sugar levels. The phytonutrient falcarinol seems to protect the colon. Carrots are considered a diuretic and are a traditional cure for water-retention. Nutrients concentrate just beneath the skin.

Carrot seed oil is valued in skin preparations for having beneficial properties that can smooth away fine lines and counter skin discoloration, such as rashes or melasma (the mask of pregnancy). However, it is best avoided until after childbirth, being used traditionally to bring on menstruation.

BUYING NOTES

Carrots should be firm—floppy ones have lost many nutrients. The deeper the carrot's color, the more beta-carotene it contains. If bunches have their feathery tops, gauge the freshness by the state of the leaves but cut off the green tops before storing to prevent moisture-loss. Buy organic; carrots have been identified as one of the 12 most pesticide-contaminated foods.

Canned carrots are also a good choice; canning makes the carotenoids easier for your body to absorb.

GROWING AND HARVESTING NOTES

Carrots can be tricky to germinate and get established. Sow very thinly to avoid the need to thin in situ, which attracts carrot fly, or sow in containers to fool the carrot fly (which travels horizontally). If they are to form good roots, carrots need a fertile, well-drained, deep and fine soil, so have someone work in lots of grit, compost, and manure the previous fall—you can do the light, regular weeding required during the growing season.

Different varieties come to maturity through the growing year, from early harvest short, squat cultivars ready in midsummer, such as Nantes, to longer and larger roots that crop the following spring, such as Chantenay, which have a fine flavor. Globe-shaped roots look attractive and suit shallower soils or container planting.

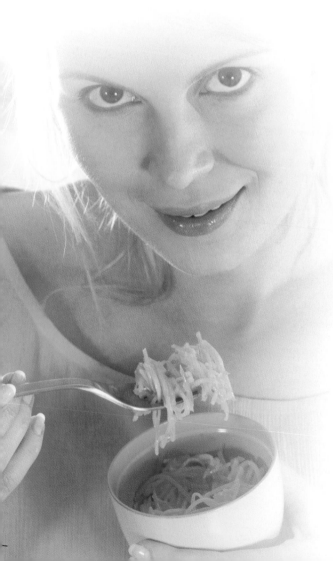

Although it's an old wives' tale that eating carrots creates a child with red hair and a fiery temper, they are vitamin-packed vegetables.

Pick carrots young—about the size of your little finger—to serve raw. Later in the season lift carefully with a fork to avoid snapping the root.

CULINARY DOS AND DON'TS

- Don't peel carrots; simply scrub them to preserve nutrients (make sure you use organic produce).
- Cook carrots to make beta-carotene more available for the body to use. Eat carrots with a little fat to aid the absorption of beta-carotene.
- Halve carrots and roast for at least 30 minutes with a joint of meat.

QUICK AND EASY DISHES

- *Combine shredded carrot with warm, toasted sunflower seeds dressed with a little balsamic vinegar.*
- *Grate a little organic orange zest over cooked carrots before serving.*

GINGER

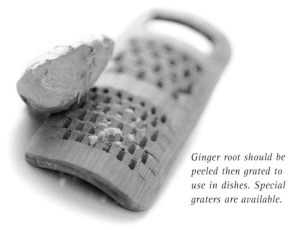

The word "zingy" derives from the botanical name for ginger, *Zingiber officinale*, and this is just the thing to pep up flagging energy levels and shake nausea from your system. Research on pregnant women has shown that ginger is both safe and effective at alleviating the symptoms of morning sickness—even the most severe types. Keep ginger cookies or gingersnaps by the bed and drink ginger ale when your spirits need lifting.

The fresh root has higher amounts of beneficial properties than the dried powder. Sticky candied ginger, cooked in a sugar syrup, is a treat in tiny amounts. Ginger syrup is handy for sweetening tea. When choosing ginger cordial, look for products cold pressed from fresh ginger root.

Ginger root should be peeled then grated to use in dishes. Special graters are available.

GOOD FOR YOU AND BABY

Ginger contains good amounts of potassium, magnesium, copper, manganese, and vitamin B_6. Its anti-nausea properties stem from the ingredient that gives the distinctive zingy taste: the pungent phenolic compound gingerol, which is highly antioxidant and has analgesic and antibacterial properties. Protease makes ginger anti-inflammatory.

Many studies show just how effective ginger is at preventing travel sickness, and several have found it more effective than a placebo in controlling pregnancy nausea and vomiting. Ginger is also a traditional cold cure. Herbalists treating pregnant women might recommend ginger to counter constipation and gas, quell cramping, tone the pelvic muscles, soothe the digestive tract and aid digestion.

The optimum amount for pregnancy vomiting is 250 mg taken 4 times daily. Consult your doctor if you are taking blood-thinning medication. Since ginger seems to help prevent blood clotting, it may be best to stop using it in the weeks leading up to birth.

BUYING NOTES

When buying fresh ginger root, snap off a section and check that it's juicy and not too fibrous. The skin should have a sheen. Avoid wrinkled specimens.

QUICK AND EASY DISHES

- *To make fresh ginger tea, grate ½–1 inch of root into a mug and pour over boiling water; steep for 5 minutes and sweeten with honey. To combat a cold or chill, add a squeeze of fresh lemon.*

ginger

🌱 BLACK CURRANTS AND RASPBERRIES

Currants and berries may be the most delicious instant snacks there are. It's best to eat them fresh because many of the health benefits derive from the phenolic compounds anthocyanins, which are destroyed during processing. Black currants, however, are rarely eaten raw as they are very acidic. Unlike raspberries, they are not ubiquitous in supermarkets. You may need to source them from farmers' markets or grow at home. Red and white currants are sweeter varieties of the same plant.

Red raspberry leaf tea (see page 35) is the best-known herbal pregnancy tonic, recommended to strengthen the uterus during pregnancy and restore your health following the birth of your child.

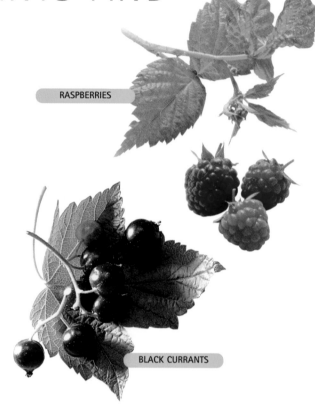

RASPBERRIES

BLACK CURRANTS

GOOD FOR YOU AND YOUR BABY

Both black currants and raspberries are rich in vitamin C; there is more in a few black currants than in a whole lemon. Raspberries are high in manganese and contain B vitamins and folate, too. Both are great sources of fiber. Black currants have more potassium than bananas and are one of the few plant sources of the essential fatty acid gamma-linolenic acid.

The extreme antioxidant activity in raspberries is a result of ellagitannins and the flavonoid molecules anthocyanins, which are responsible also for the color and for the berries' antimicrobial and anti-inflammatory properties. Frozen raspberries have similar antioxidant properties to fresh. The oil of red raspberry seeds contains vitamin E and omega-3 fatty acids, and protects the skin against the sun.

Red raspberry leaves are rich in iron and are commonly used during the third trimester to tone the uterine and pelvic muscles, making contractions more effective. They are also recommended by herbalists to combat nausea and bleeding gums and ease labor pain. After childbirth, the leaves are recommended to speed healing and boost milk production. In an Australian study, mothers who took a 1.2 g tablet daily from 32 weeks had a shorter second stage and reduced risk of a forceps delivery. Other research associates use with a reduced risk of delivering early or late.

Many midwives advise women not to use the herb without a herbalist's advice until week 36. Then it seems safe to build up from 1 to 3–4 cups of red raspberry leaf tea a day and to sip it through labor.

BUYING NOTES

Avoid punnets containing mushy, over-ripe or moldy currants or berries. Raspberries don't travel well; those grown locally are likely to be riper and better textured.

GROWING AND HARVESTING NOTES

Grow black currants as a bush if you feel lazy; if you feel like doing more work, train them onto a trellis or fence, which can look spectacular and makes for easier picking when you can't bend forward. Plant currants and raspberries during the dormant winter months, cutting back the stems to promote new growth. Manure and mulch in the spring.

Of the Rubus (raspberry) species, the garden cultivar is the European red raspberry *Rubus idaeus*, whereas the variety thought to be valued through history for its uterine toning is the wild American red raspberry *Rubus strigosus*. *R. idaeus* has been shown in tests to contain caffeic acid, which can suppress pregnancy hormones, and has been associated with spotting and miscarriage. For this reason it is not recommended by many midwives in the first trimester.

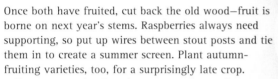

Once both have fruited, cut back the old wood—fruit is borne on next year's stems. Raspberries always need supporting, so put up wires between stout posts and tie them in to create a summer screen. Plant autumn-fruiting varieties, too, for a surprisingly late crop.

Protect canes by throwing over netting so that you, rather than the birds, can harvest the fruit. Berries are ready to pick when they come away easily from the white core. Eat immediately. Reserve those past their best for jelly-making.

CULINARY DOS AND DON'TS

- Toss currants and berries into breakfast cereal and oatmeal.
- Crush and stir into yogurt or use to fill pancakes.
- Make jelly from black currants to temper their tartness.
- Serve a red currant sauce to cut through the richness of venison or oily fish.

RASPBERRY LEAF TEA

If you find the taste of this tea too astringent, substitute half the amount of raspberry leaves with an equal amount of rosehip or lemon balm. Many medical practitioners advise that you don't drink this tea until the third trimester.

    1 oz dried red raspberry leaves
    Honey, to taste

Place the leaves in a teapot and pour over 2 cups of just-boiled water. Allow to steep for 10 minutes. Strain into a cup and sweeten to taste with the honey. To reserve the tea for later, once cold, strain into a container, cover, and refrigerate. Warm up or drink cold.

MORNING SICKNESS CORDIAL

Vitamins C and K have been shown to be valuable in easing morning sickness. Try this cordial when you wake. Black currants, strawberries, and kiwifruit are high in vitamin C, while kiwifruit contains moderate amounts of vitamin K and strawberries are rich in folate.

    1½ cups strawberries
    2 ripe kiwifruit
    1 cup black currants
    1⅓ cups caster sugar

Remove the leaves from the strawberries, peel and slice the kiwi, and top and tail the currants. Place all the fruit in a large pan with the sugar and 4 cups water and bring to boil. Then turn down the heat and simmer, stirring, for 5–10 minutes, or until the fruit has broken down and the liquid is reduced. Pour into a strainer over a bowl and press the fruit pulp with the back of a wooden spoon to extract as much juice and pulp as you can. Decant into a sterilized bottle. Lid and allow to cool. Refrigerate until ready to use. Dilute a little cordial with cold, hot or carbonated water, to taste.

black currants and raspberries

SALAD GREENS

Remember the fairy tale Rapunzel? It was the pregnant wife's craving for fresh green lettuce leaves that kickstarted the action. Old stories are often based on truths. Perhaps lettuces seem so lush and moreish as our bellies swell because they contain a blend of vitamins, minerals, and phytonutrients that supports a healthy pregnancy. In China, eating plenty of lettuce in the days before conception is thought to build a boy. In British lore, it is considered an aid to conception. If you're having trouble sleeping, eat a lettuce salad or sandwich before bed: the leaves contain a known soporific.

GOOD FOR YOU AND YOUR BABY

A rich source of vitamins A, B, C, K and folate, with good amounts of manganese, chromium, potassium, and iron, lettuce also contains calcium and omega-3 fatty acids, fiber, and protein. Loose-leaf lettuces contain more nutrients, since the leaves have opened to the light. Red-colored leaves, such as Lollo Rossa, contain the antioxidant flavonol quertecin. In one study, women who ate lettuce daily seemed to have stronger bones.

BUYING NOTES

The shorter the journey from soil to plate, the tastier this plant will be. Look for lettuce at farm shops. Favor deep green, crispy, juicy-looking leaves and avoid those with oxidized browning or yellow discoloration. Lettuce wrapped in plastic in supermarkets will be deficient in vitamin B_{12}. Buy organic to be sure the leaves have not been sprayed: lettuce is one of the worst foods for pesticide residue.

Lettuce divide into hearted and nonhearting varieties. The hearted include deep green butterheads, which are soft, blowsy, and tasty; crispheads, which tend to be tasteless and color-free; and romaine (or cos), which are both flavorful and stand up to handling. Then there are the nonhearting, or loose-leaf, lettuces, which include oak-leaved type salad bowls, curly lollos, and catalogna, which have elongated, arrow-shaped serrated leaves. Soft butterhead varieties wilt sooner than ball-shaped crispheads, which are easier to transport and keep longer, so form a tasteless supermarket staple.

GROWING AND HARVESTING NOTES

Grow your own soft-hearted and cut-and-come-again lettuces, which don't travel well to supermarkets. Sow

---

QUICK AND EASY DISHES

- *Make a vinaigrette with one part balsamic to six parts olive oil; add a squeeze of lemon, sea salt and black pepper, a touch of grainy mustard and honey, then shake or beat to combine. Pour over lettuce.*

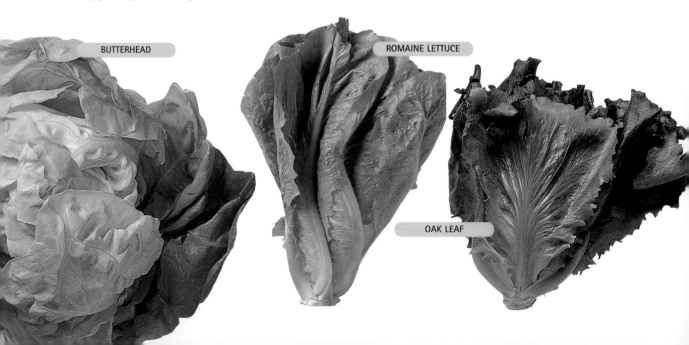

BUTTERHEAD

ROMAINE LETTUCE

OAK LEAF

fortnightly into light, fertile soil for a successional crop and to prevent bolting—try grow bags or the front of a raised bed. Be vigilant in your watch for slugs and snails, and snack on the thinnings.

Pick and eat the same day. Pull romaine or round lettuces whole. Loose-leaf types can be used as cut-and-come-again crops (see page 40)—either harvest a few leaves at once or cut off above the lowest leaves, then leave the plant to regrow.

CULINARY DOS AND DON'TS
- Don't cut leaves; tear them to prevent wilting and oxidization (and nutrient loss).
- Pat leaves dry before tossing in dressing so the dressing sticks to the leaves rather than the bowl.
- Combine lettuce with asparagus and peas as a salad to maximize folate.
- If nausea masks your hunger, start a meal with a little lettuce; it is thought to stimulate the appetite.
- Serve crunchy romaine leaves as a scoop for dips.

MUSTARD GREENS

If you crave salad in winter, avoid the midwinter fresh greens gap (and floppy supermarket offerings) by eating Asian leaves: Komatsuna, or mustard greens, have an intense, fiery, spinach-type flavor that can stimulate a jaded palate. Mizuna tastes more mustardy, while land cress tastes as pungently peppery and is as nutrient-filled as watercress.

GOOD FOR YOU AND YOUR BABY
Packed with vitamins C and K and beta-carotene, mustard greens also contain folate, manganese, vitamins B_6 and E, and magnesium. These leaves also contain calcium, which, when packaged with vitamin B_6 and folate as here, promotes bone health. Mustard greens are brassicas and share many of their benefits during pregnancy (see page 15), but when served raw they have more folate than broccoli.

In English lore the seeds of mustard plants are thought to encourage conception, while in Bangladesh they are scattered outside the labor room to ward off any ill-wishers.

BUYING NOTES
Mustard greens are widely available at farmers' markets and in winter organic vegetable boxes. Choose dark-colored leaves and avoid any that are yellowing or spotted. Ask the supplier if you can taste a little before buying if you don't tolerate heat well during pregnancy.

GROWING AND HARVESTING NOTES
Sow in late summer and early autumn for winter picking, and keep the plants well watered as they grow to prevent bolting. Sow again in early spring for a follow-on crop. Mustard greens do best on sunny south-facing windowsills.

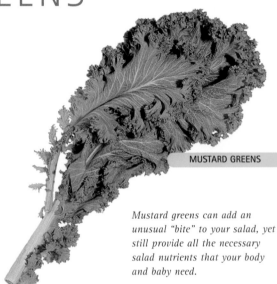

MUSTARD GREENS

Mustard greens can add an unusual "bite" to your salad, yet still provide all the necessary salad nutrients that your body and baby need.

Treat as cut-and-come-again crops (see page 40), cutting away above the lower leaves and leaving the plants to resprout over and again until spring. Or pick individual leaves as and when you fancy a snack. Mizuna grows in mustardy sharpness the longer it is in the ground.

CULINARY DOS AND DON'TS
- Use the young leaves in salads and sandwiches; add the older leaves to stir-fries.
- When using in salads, cut away and discard the central stem.
- Substitute land cress for watercress in salads and soups.
- Serve cooked mustard greens as a side dish with spicy beans and rice.

mustard greens

✿ TOMATOES

Many studies attest to the benefits of tomatoes for cardiovascular and eye health, but in one 2004 Indian study, pregnant women who ate tomato extract daily from early in pregnancy had a lower risk of pre-eclampsia and their babies grew well. (The daily amount of lycopene was the equivalent of 1 tbsp tomato sauce.)

Despite the range of tomatoes on sale at the supermarket, it's impossible to replicate the taste of a homegrown tomato picked from the vine while warm from the sun. It is easy to plant cherry tomatoes in a hanging basket outside your window, or in pots beside the door so you can start the day by inhaling the uplifting aroma of the leaves. Like other fruit with multiple seeds, tomatoes are considered a fertility-boosting food in many traditions.

If you crave tomatoes, start the day with a glass of tomato-rich vegetable juice. If you like ketchup, buy organic; in studies it contained three times as much lycopene as the non-organic variety.

GOOD FOR YOU AND YOUR BABY

Tomatoes are extremely rich in vitamin C and contain good amounts of beta-carotene, vitamin K, potassium, and manganese; they also supply B vitamins and folate, copper and iron, fiber, and some protein. Tomatoes are the primary dietary source of the antioxidant carotenoid lycopene, which protects DNA from oxygen damage, is anti-inflammatory, and supports a healthy heart. In one study, women with the highest intake of tomato-based foods had the most reduced risk of heart disease. Lycopene is most potent in cooked tomatoes, and tomato paste is one of the best sources.

BUYING NOTES

Tomatoes that have traveled less far tend to have more taste because they can be picked ripe, though new breeds of cherry or cherry plum tomato have been bred to be extra sweet and flavorful. The redder the tomatoes, the more lycopene they contain. Plum tomatoes are best for cooking since they have more flesh to juice and fewer seeds. At farmers' markets look for yellow, orange, pink and striped heirloom varieties, and odd-shaped fruit, such as the ribbed Marmande.

Check the "spidery" calyx for freshness; it should look green and alive. Outside peak harvest season—late summer to early fall—it's hard to find full-flavored tomatoes. Substitute with canned plum tomatoes, which have been picked ripe (try San Marzano or other Italian-canned brands). Sun-dried tomatoes preserved in olive oil are a good winter staple.

GROWING AND HARVESTING NOTES

Tomatoes are easy to grow if you have a long, light, warm summer. Bush varieties suit small spaces and

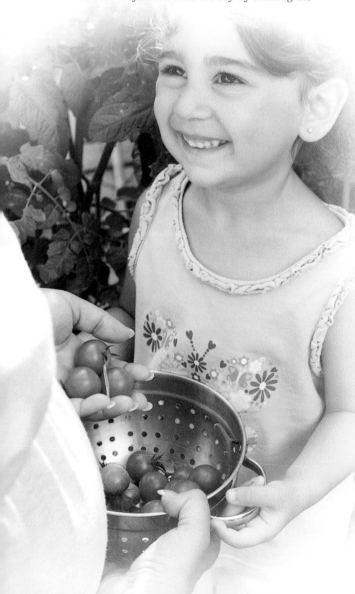

The redder the tomatoes, the more lycopene they contain.

don't require staking, nipping, or stopping. Dwarf types are also good for containers. The larger the container, the better chance of a good crop—limit grow bags to two plants each.

Cherry tomatoes are easiest to crop outdoors in cooler climates. Tumbling varieties don't need staking and do well in containers and hanging baskets. Don't overwater while the fruit are swelling; the best-flavored benefit from arid Mediterranean conditions.

Pick when fully ripe. Toward the end of the season, if fruit are semiripe, cut down the plant and hang so the tomatoes ripen indoors.

CULINARY DOS AND DON'TS
- Eat the seeds; nutrients concentrate in the jelly-like substance around them.
- Don't peel the skin—lycopene is found here.
- Crush canned plum tomatoes between your fingers—the Italian way—instead of chopping.
- To bring out the flavor of less-than-ripe tomatoes, add 1 tsp brown sugar.

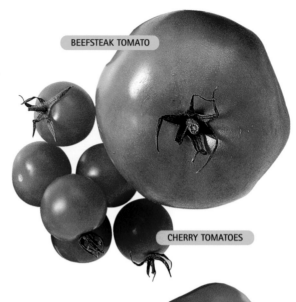

BEEFSTEAK TOMATO

CHERRY TOMATOES

PLUM TOMATO

SALAD TOMATOES

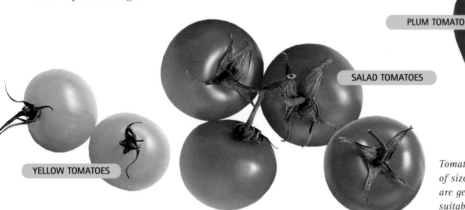

YELLOW TOMATOES

Tomatoes come in a vast array of sizes and different types but are generally divided into those suitable for slicing or cooking. Green tomatoes are pickled and plum tomatoes used for sauces.

QUICK AND EASY DISHES
- *Slice ripe tomatoes and serve dressed with a fruity olive oil, sea salt and black pepper, and torn fresh basil leaves.*
- *To make fresh tomato sauce from truly ripe tomatoes, just chop, place in a pan, put on the lid and allow to steam for around 15 minutes. Can be frozen in portions.*
- *Roast fresh whole tomatoes, quartered onions, and garlic cloves for 15–20 minutes, then stir into pasta or couscous, or spread on toast.*

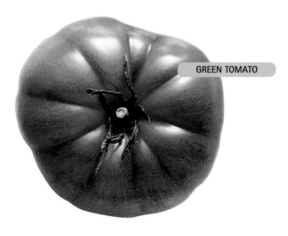

GREEN TOMATO

tomatoes

CUT-AND-COME-AGAIN CRATE

Having a fresh and constant supply of fruit and vegetables is important for supplying the vitamins, minerals, and plant nutrients you need more of in pregnancy, such as vitamin C and folate. Nor do you need to have a garden; an amazing amount of produce can be harvested year-round from planters, window boxes, and balconies—from salad greens for summer and winter to garlic and even lemons.

Plant a variety of lettuces and harvest a few leaves from each for a daily mixed-leaf salad. If you plant in a crate, you can bring it to the table to harvest. A supermarket or vegetable delivery box or a wooden orange crate has ready-made drainage holes. For constant cropping, plant a new crate every 2–3 weeks, from late winter to late spring.

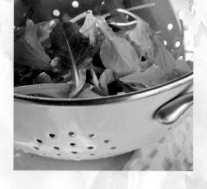

For a good combination of tastes and textures, you will need the following seeds:

Frilly loose-leaf lettuce, such as Lollo Rosso
Oak-leafed Salad Bowl
Stiff-leafed miniature semi-romaine, such as Little Gem.

1 Put on gloves. Fill the bottom and sides of the crate with heavy-duty plastic, cutting drainage holes in the bottom. Fill almost to the top with compost from a grow bag. Flatten down with your hands to remove air pockets. Water.

2 Sow the seeds thinly directly into the damp soil in rows about 4 inches apart. Alternate the varieties. Cover with a layer of dry soil. Keep in a cool place until they have germinated (by late spring the soil may be too warm for germination).

3 Thin out the seedlings when they reach about 2 inches and have 4–5 leaves (either eat them or try transplanting into another crate). Water the soil daily, if necessary, trying to avoid the foliage.

4 After 3–4 weeks, start cutting the leaves to eat, when the plants reach 2–4 inches in height. Either cut the whole head or individual leaves. The lettuces should resprout two or even three times. The loose-leaf lettuce will come up first and the romaine last.

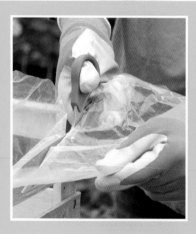

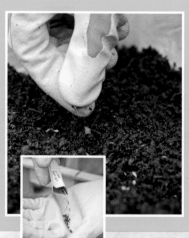

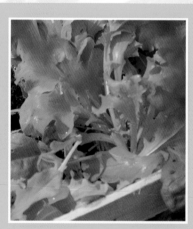

PRESERVING TOMATOES

To preserve a glut of tomatoes, roast in a slow oven before freezing in meal-size batches. You'll be glad of the supply once your baby is here. This process concentrates the flavors of summer while adding a sweet caramelized richness, and doesn't require time-consuming sterilizing.

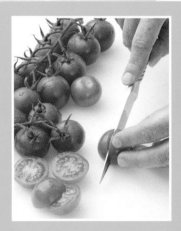

1 Preheat the oven to 284°F. Rinse the tomatoes, pat dry then pull off the vine. Remove the calyx and cut in half.

2 Place the tomatoes on baking sheets in a single layer, cut-side up, and sprinkle with a little sea salt, brown sugar, black pepper, and dried oregano. Drizzle with extra-virgin olive oil.

3 Place in the oven for 2–3 hours. The tomatoes are ready when shrunk to about two-thirds their original size. They should be dried, but still moist.

4 Once cool, divide into zip-lock bags labeled with the name and date. Spoon into each bag enough for a family meal, then freeze. To use, defrost, then stir into pasta or warm salads, or use to top crusty bread.

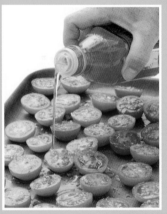

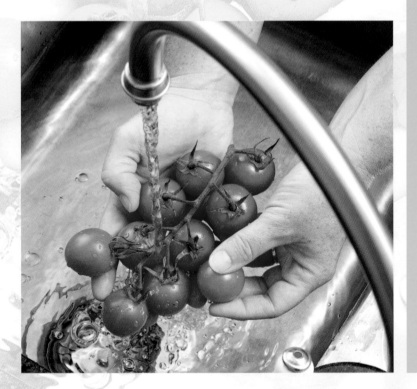

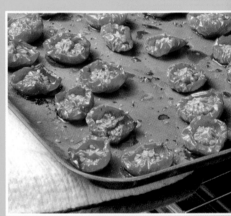

GARLIC

An ancient Egyptian medical treatise written around 1550 BCE makes the earliest link between garlic and pregnancy, citing it as useful in childbirth. Garlic was valued by ancient Greek midwives, too, for warding off infection, healing wounds, and building strength. Today, a daily dose of garlic is recommended during pregnancy to keep away colds and infection and help prevent varicose veins and cystitis. Two to four cloves a day is the optimum adult dose. Add daily to cooking.

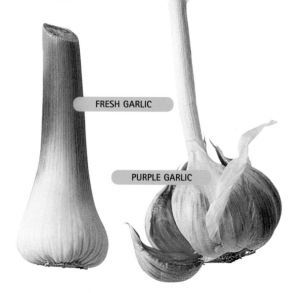

FRESH GARLIC

PURPLE GARLIC

GOOD FOR YOU AND YOUR BABY

Excellent for manganese, and a good source of vitamins B_6 and C, selenium, calcium, and phosphorus, garlic also contains protein and boosts vitamin absorption. The constituents responsible for the pungent odor—organosulfur compounds including allicin, alliin, and ajoene—also account for the numerous health benefits. They relax and enlarge the walls of blood vessels and improve blood flow, while acting as an anticoagulant, reducing the risk of varicose veins as well as of heart attack and stroke. Garlic also seems to act similarly to "good" HDL cholesterol, reducing arterial plaque.

Garlic has an anti-inflammatory effect, and allicin, which emerges when cloves are crushed or cut, is a potent antimicrobial, antibacterial, antiviral, and antifungal—it guards against colds, stomach bugs and thrush, and has even been shown to thwart antibiotic-resistant bacteria, including MRSA. In one study, people who took garlic had significantly fewer colds during the winter months than those who took a placebo, and their symptoms disappeared more quickly. Garlic makes a good cough treatment and decongestant. Some studies suggest that garlic can help combat fatigue.

Reduce your intake of garlic in the weeks before delivery to prevent excessive bleeding due to its blood-thinning properties.

BUYING NOTES

Press the heads; they should be hard and the skin unbroken. Discard those that are soft or sprouted. Buy new season pink garlic when you see it; it's a real treat. Processed garlic products from health stores do not have the health benefits of the raw cloves.

GROWING AND HARVESTING NOTES

For container planting, choose deep pots at least 6 inches wide. In early–late fall, break plump cloves from a bulb and press each one about $1\frac{1}{2}$ inches into well-drained potting compost, pointy end up (one clove per pot). Then forget about them (water if dry). The bulbs like the cold and send up fresh green stems through the winter.

Bulbs are ready to harvest from midsummer, when the leaves start to yellow, but you can cut and eat the green shoots from spring. Early harvest bulbs—"green" or "wet" garlic—are especially succulent and pungent. When digging up, work around the bulbs carefully with a fork so they come up in one piece. Leave in a sunny place outside to dry for around a week, or hang indoors in an airy place. To braid bulbs for hanging, moisten the leaves and weave together.

CULINARY DOS AND DON'TS

- The green tops of growing garlic can be cut and used in salads or as you would chives.
- Wait for a few minutes after chopping or crushing cloves before using them to allow the maximum release of allicin.
- Garlic is most antibacterial raw: crush into vinaigrettes with balsamic vinegar and honey.
- To bring out the natural sweetness, throw whole cloves in a roasting pan for 30 minutes. Squeeze out the oozing puree onto toast.
- If you find raw garlic fiery, poach in a little water or milk before use to temper the flavor.
- Don't microwave garlic; this destroys its blood-thinning properties.

QUICK AND EASY DISHES
- *Crush a few cloves and mash with an anchovy fillet and olive oil; spread onto bread and broil.*

SCALLIONS AND CHIVES

SCALLIONS

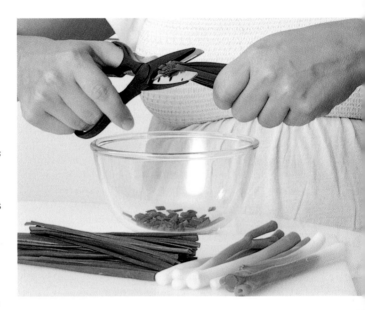

Scallions are simply young onions that have been harvested before the bulb has swollen and while the stems are still green and fresh.

The onion family raises the nutritional and health status of any meal and is helpful in keeping away coughs and colds. Scallions or green onions are valued more for their leaves than their tiny bulbs. Chinese chives are thicker and more pungently garlicky than regular chives. Since medieval times and in various cultures onions have the reputation of encouraging milk production in nursing mothers. The smaller members of the onion family are easily raised in containers.

GOOD FOR YOU AND YOUR BABY

Onions are a good source of chromium and vitamin C and also supply manganese, vitamin B_6, potassium, folate, potassium, phosphorus, and copper. The onion family is a good fiber food. The constituent flavonoid quercetin protects the digestive tract and has antioxidant and anti-inflammatory actions.

Many of the benefits of garlic (see opposite page) also apply to onions, since they share antimicrobial, antibacterial, and anticoagulant organosulfur compounds. These are not lost during cooking. Onion also stimulates the gastric juices, benefiting digestion, and seems to lower blood-sugar levels.

BUYING NOTES

Choose firm scallion bulbs with crisp green leaves. Avoid those with soft whites or yellowing tips. Sniff before you buy: the smellier varieties have more health-protecting phytonutrients.

GROWING AND HARVESTING NOTES

Scallions do well in containers as thin as lengths of guttering. They are best grown from seed in potting compost. Sow thinly every 2–3 weeks (for successive cropping) from early spring to early summer and eat the thinnings. They like a sunny site. It's easiest to buy

chives as young plants rather than growing from seed, or to divide an existing clump.

Scallions are ready to eat around 12 weeks after sowing. Ease them up with a hand fork to keep the bulb whole. To encourage the secondary growth of chives, cut them back hard after the first year and watch them sprout again.

CULINARY DOS AND DON'TS

- Chop scallions into diagonal lengths (using the leaves as well as the bulbs) to stir-fry; snip chives.
- Stir chives into potato salads and mashed potato.
- Chives add piquancy to dressings for fish and also work well with omelets.
- Use the buds and flowers from chives to decorate salads.
- Store in the salad drawer of the fridge for up to three days.

QUICK AND EASY DISHES
- *Chop scallions finely and mix with tomato, lime juice, and cilantro to make a sweet salsa.*

LEMONS

The cheerful sunshine-hue of this fruit and its citrussy freshness can't fail to lift the spirits when everything aches and you haven't seen your feet for weeks. If you're prone to nausea, start the day with a squeeze of lemon juice topped up with hot water and sweetened with honey (and possibly ginger) and keep lemon candies in your bag to suck when nausea strikes on journeys.

GOOD FOR YOU AND YOUR BABY

Lemons are one of the best sources of vitamin C and also supply potassium. Flavonoids protect DNA and have antibacterial properties, while limonoid and limonene phytochemicals stimulate the body's detoxification systems and lower cholesterol. Austrian research shows that the riper the fruit, the greater its antioxidant properties. A 1987 study suggested that drinking lemon juice boosts absorption of iron.

Essential oil of lemon may be used by aromatherapists for pregnancy massage to treat digestive problems and symptoms of stress, or as a pick-me-up. Leave treatment to a professional though; this oil is a potential skin irritant and photosensitizer.

BUYING NOTES

Choose fully ripe, thin-skinned lemons (for extra juice) that are heavy for their size. Non-waxed organic lemons are safest: they have fewer chemical coatings, which is important if you are zesting the fruit to eat. But do buy fresh, since they shrivel and decay more quickly than waxed produce. At farmers' markets keep an eye out for smaller, sweeter, more fragrant varieties such as Meyer's, a mandarin hybrid, and for specialties such as the super-tangy Sicilian or sweet swollen Sorrento lemons.

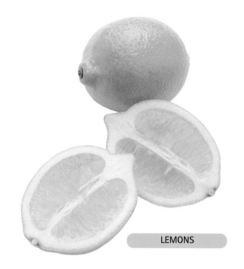

LEMONS

The smell of lemons freshly cut is said by some to relieve morning sickness (or try two drops of essential oil of lemon on a tissue).

GROWING NOTES

Lemon trees can be bought in pots with blossom and lemons already growing. In cooler climates, make sure your container can winter indoors or under glass. Lemon trees require ericaceous compost (acidic soil with a pH less than 7), watering, and good drainage. To keep the foliage glossy and the colorful fruit on the tree, feed through the winter with a plant food rich in trace elements. Repot in a large container as the tree grows.

Resist the temptation to pick the fruit until it is fully ripe. The heady perfume of the blossom is as much a treat in winter as the fruit.

CULINARY DOS AND DON'TS

- To extract maximum juice, warm the fruit between your palms.
- Use the zest, a concentrated source of limonoids and limonenes. When zesting, be careful not to pare off the white pith below, which is bitter.
- Try a squeeze of lemon as a flavor enhancer for fish and chickpea dishes.
- Use lemon juice to prevent cut fruit such as apples or artichokes from oxidizing.
- If you can find large Sorrento lemons, slice finely and serve as an accompaniment to grilled meat, with a drizzle of good olive oil and a sprinkling of sea salt.

QUICK AND EASY DISHES

- *Add lemon juice to sparkling mineral water to act as a healthy alternative to carbonated drinks.*
- *Mix lemon juice with olive oil, garlic, fresh marjoram, and salt and pepper and use to marinate chicken or ground lamb.*
- *Combine lemon juice and olive oil to make a light salad dressing.*

STRAWBERRIES AND BLUEBERRIES

With more vitamin C than lemons, strawberries make perfect pregnancy treats. In one study (reported in *Epidemiology*), pregnant women who ate lots of vitamin C rich foods had a lower risk of pre-eclampsia. Blueberries are also incredibly healthy during pregnancy. In tests, cultivated blueberries were ranked fourth most antioxidant fruit or vegetable (wild ones ranked number two), more potent than red wine.

GOOD FOR YOU AND YOUR BABY

Strawberries and blueberries are an excellent source of vitamin C and also supply manganese. Strawberries add iodine and potassium, superb amounts of folate, plus B vitamins, omega-3 fatty acids, magnesium, and copper, while blueberries offer vitamin E. Both strawberries and blueberries are good sources of fiber. The phenolic compounds, anthocyanins, are responsible for the rich color of these berries and their cell-protecting antioxidant properties. Just 20 strawberries is enough to register raised antioxidant activity in the blood. Phenols also have an anti-inflammatory action.

Blueberries support the vascular system, the ellagic acid and pectin within them also contribute to gastrointestinal health. Their tannins boost the health of the urinary tract, too, preventing infection in a similar way to cranberries.

During pregnancy (and before conceiving, if possible), become a strawberry lover. A single serving of 8 medium berries provides nearly 9 percent of the daily requirement of folate.

BUYING NOTES

Monster strawberries tend to be tasteless. For real flavor, look for old-fashioned Alpine or woodland varieties, which are tiny but intense in the mouth.

Though available year-round, nothing beats a fragrant strawberry picked in season locally. Look for pick-your-own farms. Buy to eat rather than store. Avoid punnets with a single moldy or soft fruit; green fruit will always taste sour. Buy organic as strawberries are among the most likely pesticide-contaminated foods. Ripe blueberries are a dark puplish-black; those tinged red or green will taste sour. This fruit wrinkles with age, so choose plump, smooth berries.

Bear in mind that frozen blueberries are the best source of nutrients outside your local harvest season.

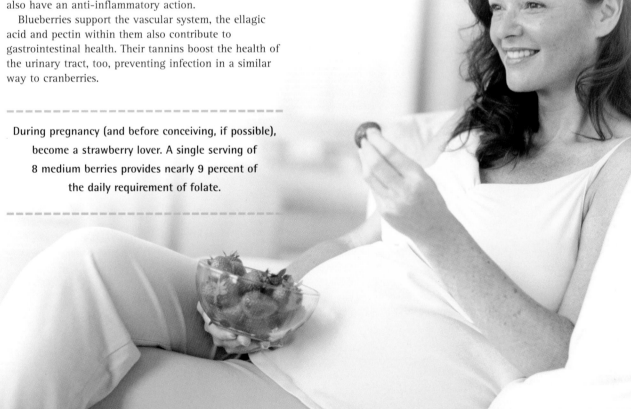

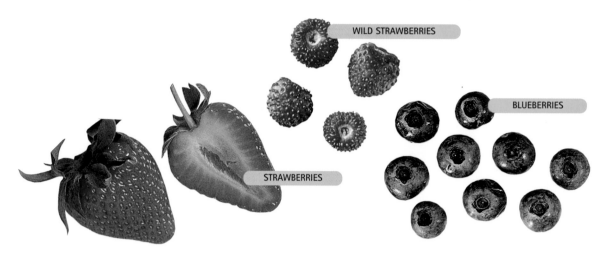

WILD STRAWBERRIES

BLUEBERRIES

STRAWBERRIES

GROWING AND HARVESTING NOTES

Strawberries are so easy to grow in containers that there is a special pot for the purpose. Make sure the soil is rich and the position sunny. Strawberry pots are designed to keep the fruit off the soil. Start with a layer of crocks (see page 18), then fill with potting compost to the first level of holes. Add a plant to pop out of each hole. Fill with more compost to the next layer and repeat until you reach the top. Site in a sunny place and keep watered. Blueberries like ericaceous soil and large pots; again, keep the soil moist. Prune out dead and nonfruiting older (darker) branches in the winter.

For a constant supply of berries, plant early and late fruiting varieties. Self-pollinating blueberries are essential if you don't have room for different cultivars. Plants are very productive; you can pick berries off them for weeks.

Pick strawberries when just ripe or the birds will get them. Blueberries are less attractive to birds, but CDs tied to the bush do deter. Blueberries are ready when they are dark, firm and have a silver bloom.

CULINARY DOS AND DON'TS

- Eat berries raw—anthocyanins are lost during all processing except freezing—and as fresh as you can; storage depletes folate and vitamin C.
- The riper the berry, the higher the antioxidant levels.
- If you know the source and trust that the blueberries are organic and home-grown, don't wash them as this is damaging.
- Enhance the flavor of strawberries with a grating of black pepper.
- Add a squeeze of lemon to intensify the fruity flavors of berries.

LABOR-ENERGY DRINK

Blueberries are a native American species, and Native Americans brewed a tea from the root to speed childbirth. Don't try this with your own roots; they are unlikely to be of the right species. Instead, sip this sweet cordial during labor to maintain energy and stave off dehydration, nausea, and headaches.

2 cups blueberries
juice of ½ lemon
1–2 tbsp honey

Destalk the blueberries and put them in a pan. Cook over low heat until they give up their juice. Whiz in a blender, add the lemon juice and honey, checking for sweetness (add more honey if necessary) and serve over crushed ice, topped up with water, to taste.

QUICK AND EASY DISHES

- *Whiz strawberries with yogurt and banana for a breakfast smoothie.*
- *Blend blueberries with creamy Greek yogurt and seeds from a vanilla bean.*
- *Fold berries into pancakes and use them to top waffles.*

goodnesds from the garden

46

MAKING A GINGER SYRUP

In traditional Chinese, Indian, and Arabic medicine, this root has been valued as a treatment for nausea and vomiting since ancient times—and modern clinical trials have proven it to be effective and safe in pregnancy. Adding a little of this sweet syrup to a drink or breakfast dish is a delicious way to take the cure. You will need a sterilized bottle with a lid.

You will need:

8 oz fresh ginger root
1 unwaxed organic lemon
1 cup firmly packed brown sugar

1 Wash the ginger, then grate the root finely into a large pan (don't bother to peel it). Zest the lemon into the pan, then squeeze in the juice. Add the sugar and 3 cups water.

2 Bring to a boil, stirring until the sugar has dissolved, then allow to bubble gently over medium–low heat, uncovered, for 30 minutes, until the syrup has thickened and reduced slightly.

3 Strain through cheese cloth or a fine sieve, discarding the ginger and lemon zest, then pour through a funnel into the bottle and put on the lid. Allow to cool completely, then refrigerate for up to 2 weeks.

4 To use, add a little of the syrup to hot or chilled tea (with or without milk) or pour 1–2 tablespoons into a glass and top up with sparkling water. At breakfast time, use to sweeten plain yogurt or pour over waffles or French toast.

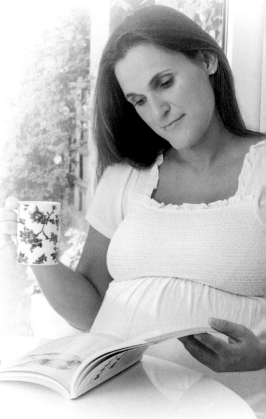

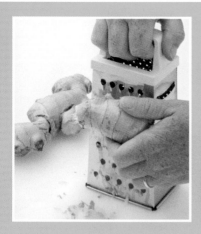
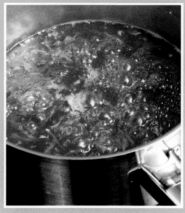
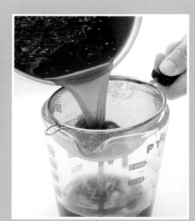

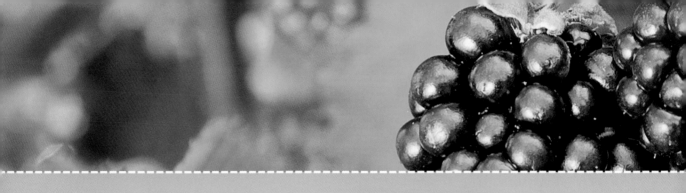
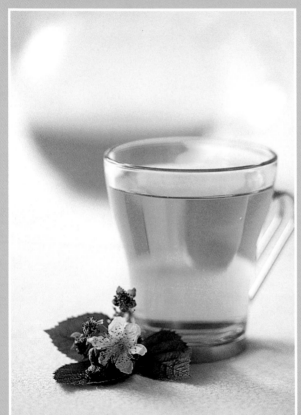
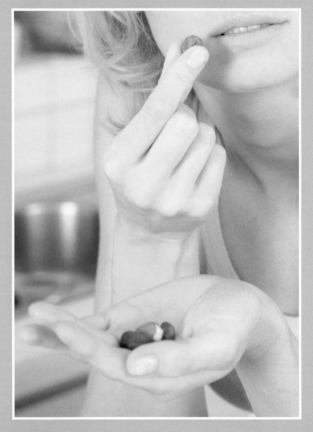
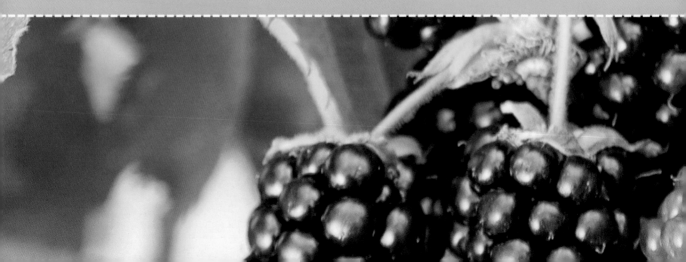

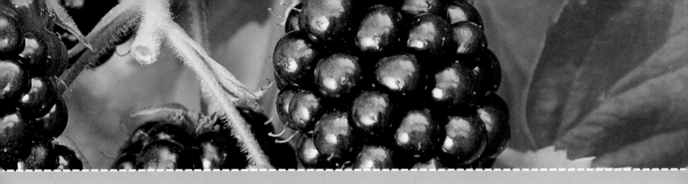

FRESH, WILD, AND FREE

Outside your door lurk free fresh foods packed with nutrients and bioactive compounds traditionally used as pregnancy tonics. So now is the time for a change of attitude: let the nettles and brambles invade and give up digging dandelions from the lawn.

NETTLES · DANDELION · HAZELNUTS · BLACKBERRIES

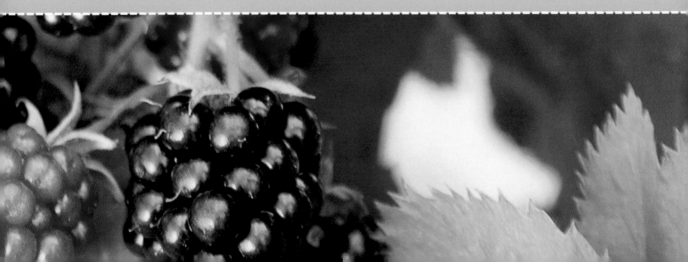

NETTLES

A neglected source of food, stinging nettles are one of nature's most nutrient-rich plants and a traditional pregnancy remedy recommended by herbalists and many midwives. However, nettles are rated by the Natural Medicines Database in the United States as "likely unsafe" for use in pregnancy, so talk to your doctor or midwife before ingesting, and consult a herbalist for specific ailments. If in doubt, reserve this valuable herb for the postpartum period, when it is useful in energizing, cleansing, and building a good supply of milk.

If you would prefer not to pick nettles yourself, look for 100 percent organic nettle tea or pregnancy tea mixes based on nettle.

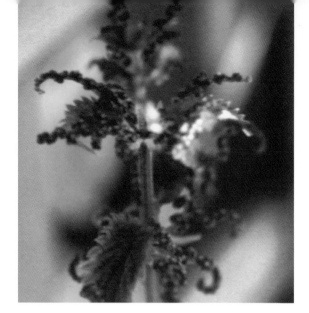

GOOD FOR YOU AND YOUR BABY

The most easily absorbed plant form of iron, nettles also contain vitamin C, which aids iron absorption. They supply potassium, calcium, and the bone-friendly beta-carotene and vitamin K, plus the trace mineral boron, which helps bones to maintain calcium. The leaves are extremely high in protein.

Nettles have diuretic properties (perhaps due to the constituent flavonoids and potassium) and can be useful for those prone to urinary tract infections or water retention. In studies, nettle tea has eased symptoms of hay fever and allergies, reduced sneezing, and soothed itchy skin. The plant can stem localized bleeding, and is used by herbalists to treat hemorrhoids and prevent hemorrhaging. It also seems to be effective in treating gastrointestinal problems. During childbirth, nettles are a traditional pain-relief medicine (affecting the way the body transmits pain impulses), and afterward are used to restore energy and increase milk production.

Never take concentrated extracts; nettles can stimulate menstruation and may contribute to miscarriage. Avoid nettles if you take blood-thinning medication or diuretics, drugs for high blood pressure or diabetes, or anti-inflammatories.

HARVESTING NOTES

Nettles grow in the same place every year. Look for the plant in spring in damp, shady places with rich soil, including near rivers. The plants can sprout new growth in the fall. The plant used medicinally is *Urtica dioica*. Recognize it by its many tiny sharp hairs on the stem and the undersides of leaves.

Pick complete young shoots in the spring (up to 6 inches tall) for use as a vegetable. For teas, pick the young leaves only (strip them downward) before the plant starts to flower some weeks later. Avoid after flowering and bypass those growing by busy roads, which might have a coating of heavy-metal laced dust. Wear thick gloves (the hairs can sting through light cotton) and snip with kitchen scissors. To dry the leaves, hang the whole stem in a dry, airy place until crispy, then store in airtight containers in a cool, dark place.

CULINARY DOS AND DON'TS
- Don't worry about the sting; it is destroyed by cooking or drying.
- Wash the leaves well to dislodge soil and bugs.
- While they are young, leave the stems on for cooking.

IRON-RICH NURSING TEA

Sip this after the birth. Nettle and rosehip are iron-rich, and rosehip's vitamin C aids its absorption. Peppermint adds taste.

1 bag organic nettle tea
1 bag organic rosehip tea
1 bag organic peppermint tea

Place the teabags in a pot and pour over 2 cups boiling water. Allow to steep for 10 minutes, then drink sweetened with honey.

- Eat young leaves only; they become bitter and fibrous with age. When chopping fresh, wear gloves.
- Steam leaves in the water from washing; adding more water destroys taste as well as nutrients.
- Use the young leaves in cooked dishes as you would spinach or kale. Try a nettle lasagna or nettle gnocchi, using a spinach recipe.
- Replace the basil in pesto with blanched, chopped nettles.
- Add a slice of lemon to nettle tea and watch the tea turn pink!

QUICK AND EASY DISHES
- *Combine with feta cheese, raisins, and pine nuts in a pastry shell.*
- *To make tea, place 1 oz of dried leaves in a teapot and pour over 2 cups boiling water; steep for 10 minutes. Or place 1 tsp dried leaves in an infuser in a mug, pour over boiling water and allow to steep for 5 minutes. Because nettle is a diuretic, accompany tea with a glass of water.*

DANDELION

Though considered an invasive pest, the nutty flavored young leaves make tasty additions to salads. You might like to try dandelion coffee if you are cutting down on regular or decaffeinated coffee.

GOOD FOR YOU AND YOUR BABY
Dandelions are a useful source of potassium, iron, calcium, zinc, beta-carotene—containing more than carrots—and vitamins B, C and D. The plant has a diuretic effect (without promoting potassium loss, like conventional medication) and is a mild laxative. Dandelion extract is used by herbalists to aid digestion, build intestinal flora, and stimulate the appetite, and can regulate blood-sugar levels. In pregnancy, it may be recommended for morning sickness and digestive complaints, but talk to your doctor or midwife before

QUICK AND EASY DISHES
- *Try fresh leaves in a thinly sliced wholemeal bread sandwich with butter, seasoning and a squeeze of lemon juice.*
- *Make a salad of fresh dandelion leaves mixed with hard-boiled egg and bacon. Toss with a warm vinaigrette.*
- *Steam the leaves and serve with garlic or a little nutmeg as a vegetable.*
- *To make tea, place 1 tsp dried leaves in an infuser in a mug, pour over boiling water and allow to steep for 5 minutes.*

ingesting it and consult a herbalist for specific ailments. The plant supports liver function and is also used to treat high blood pressure. In herbal shops, look for the botanical name *Taraxacum officinale* and organic dandelion tea bags. Because dandelion is high in vitamin A, take in moderation. Avoid if you are allergic to the daisy family or iodine.

HARVESTING NOTES
Pick the leaves for eating while young, before the plant has flowered; older leaves are tougher and more bitter.

CULINARY DOS AND DON'TS
- Wash leaves well to dislodge soil and insects.
- As with lettuces, tear the leaves to prevent the edges from oxidizing.

dandelion

HAZELNUTS

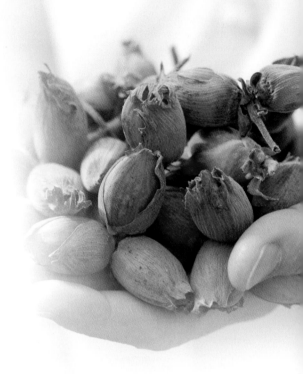

These hedgerow trees grow wild across Europe and the United States. Also known as cobnuts or filberts, hazelnuts are age-old tokens of fertility, perhaps because they are the first hedgerow plants to show signs of life in early spring and can be eaten throughout the winter. An abundance of catkins is said to augur an abundance of babies in the locality: "plenty of catkins, plenty of prams" goes an English saying. Enjoy a walk during catkin season to earmark an easy place to gather your nuts in the fall.

GOOD FOR YOU AND YOUR BABY
Hazelnuts are one of the richest sources of vitamin E, manganese, and copper, and contain impressive amounts of B vitamins and folate as well as phosphorus, magnesium, and iron. They have the most folate of any tree nut and supply protein and fiber. Hazelnuts contain proanthocyanidins—more than any other tree nut—which are associated with reduced blood clotting and infections of the urinary tract. Hazelnuts are a very good source of fat: almost 75 percent is monounsaturated, and they have one of the lowest percentages of saturated fat of any nut (less than 4 percent).

The oil is valued in massage for its fine texture and sweet scent (do a patch test if you suffer nut allergies).

HARVESTING NOTES
To get to the nuts before the squirrels, start foraging from late summer. Stroll hedgerows, keeping your eyes on the ground for fallen nuts. This is a sign that they are ready to harvest. Hook branches down with a stick for easy picking (don't go climbing ladders).

Alternatively, you may be able to find them in farmers' markets or the supermarket in summer, where they are available "in the green" and taste as moist as peas in the pod, or in the fall or midwinter when they are sold dry and hard. Green nuts have a frilly ruff around the top—the freshest look moist. Whole unshelled dried hazelnuts stay fresh longer than shelled nuts. Store these in an airtight container in a cool, dry place—light makes the fat turn rancid and moisture leads to oxidization.

CULINARY DOS AND DON'TS
- Roasting brings out the natural sweetness of hazelnuts. With skins on, spread the nuts evenly on a baking sheet and roast at 350°F for 10 minutes, shaking the the nuts occasionally. To remove the skins, which can be bitter, wrap the nuts in a dish towel for a few minutes, then rub to loosen the skins.
- Chop into muesli or use as a topping on yogurt and ice cream.
- Combine hazelnuts with dark chocolate—this is a tested taste combination (gianduja).
- Add chopped nuts to cookie and cake batters.
- Grind (or buy) as a powder to substitute for flour in cakes and to thicken winter stews and soups.

QUICK AND EASY DISHES
- *Toast the nuts and mix into a salad of young spinach leaves and sliced pear.*
- *Spice up plain cooked rice with a handful of nuts cooked with some chopped onion, mushrooms, and celery in a little butter or vegetable or hazelnut oil.*
- *Serve white or green asparagus with a dressing made of toasted and chopped hazelnuts, hazelnut oil, lemon juice, and salt and pepper. Sprinkle with grated Parmesan cheese.*

BLACKBERRIES

The ultimate food for free, blackberries grow prolifically in the wild, have an extended season, and can be more valuable for pregnancy nutrition than many cultivated superfoods or those flown from the other side of the globe. An early summer walk is a good way to spot places to pick later on—look for pink-white flowers.

Cultivated varieties don't have the flavor or tartness of taste of wild blackberries, and once picked, berries have a short shelf life (a day or so), so it's best to pick your own to eat the same day or freeze (this preserves the nutrients).

GOOD FOR YOU AND YOUR BABY

An excellent source of vitamins C and E, beta-carotene, potassium, and calcium, blackberries contain more folate than most fruit, second only to strawberries. They are one of the highest in fiber, too (up to 20 percent by weight). The purple-black color indicates the presence of anthocyanin pigments, one of the many phenolic compounds in the fruit (blackberries have the most of any berry). They also supply antiviral and antibacterial ellagic acid, which survives cooking. These potent antioxidants are good for vascular health and have anti-inflammatory properties.

Blackberry cordial is a traditional remedy for sore throats and respiratory ailments, and a tea of the leaves is used by First Nations tribes to prevent vomiting.

HARVESTING NOTES

The fruit is ready from mid-late summer until surprisingly late into the fall. A berry is ripe when it separates easily from the white core. Always wear thick gloves and long sleeves for protection from prickles.

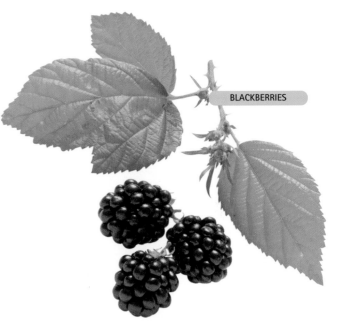

BLACKBERRIES

A member of the rose family, blackberries are among the most beneficial foods for a pregnancy diet.

CULINARY DOS AND DON'TS

- The first berry on the spur is best for eating; use subsequent ones for cooking and the last ones for jelly-making.
- When making preserves and jellies, add a pectin-rich fruit such as apples, lemons, and raspberries, to aid setting.
- Make a cordial from blackberries steeped in cider vinegar to combat colds and sore throats.
- Cooking does not destroy the vitamin E or fiber, so use liberally in puddings and jellies.
- Combine the tartness to good effect with apples.
- Freeze in small bags—enough for one crumble or pie to reprise the scents (and nutrients) of harvest season in midwinter.

QUICK AND EASY DISHES

- *Put hulled and halved blackberries in a blender and puree. Rub puree through a fine sieve set over a bowl to remove seeds. Add confectioners' sugar to taste and use to top ice creams or pancakes .*
- *Fold lightly sweetened blackberries and broken meringues into whipped cream for a quick dessert.*
- *Simmer a handful of blackberries in red wine or port and a little honey to use as a sauce.*

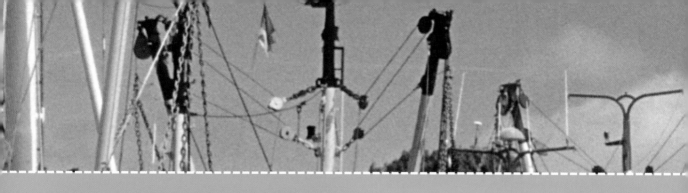

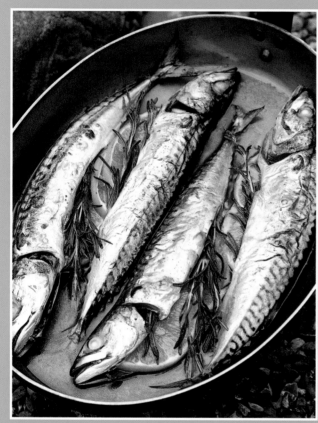

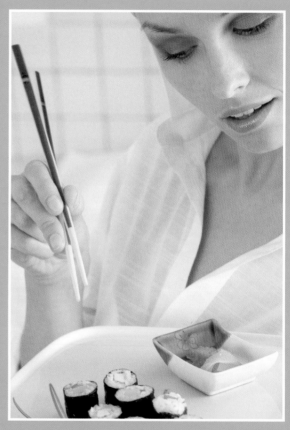

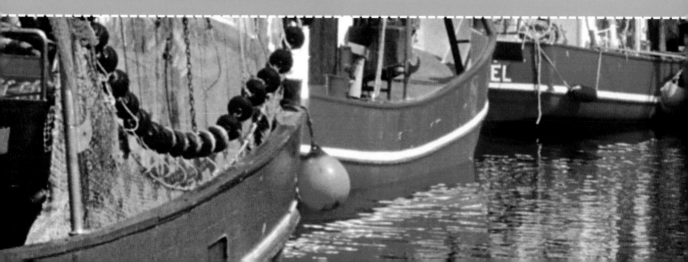

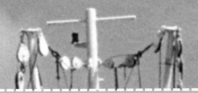

BENEFITS FROM LAKE AND SEA

Fish and other seafood are especially beneficial during pregnancy, being rich in omega-3 fatty acids—the building blocks of your baby's brain, eyes, and nervous system. Another product of the seashore—seaweed is useful for its rich mix of vitamins and minerals, including iodine, also important for brain development. Make friends with a fish merchant, the best source of information on which fish make good eating from month to month, and how to prepare them. Or look into fish box deliveries—the hassle-free way from hook to plate.

OILY FISH • SEAFOOD • SEAWEED

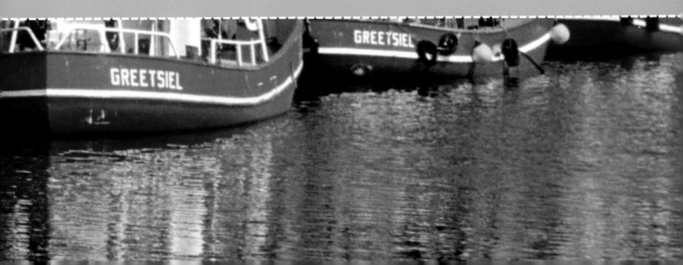

OILY FISH

The babies of mothers who eat plenty of fish during pregnancy are more likely to be brainy, studies show. These babies tend to sleep well, too, and their moms recover quickly from the birth and feel happy. You may have heard scare stories about pollutants in fish: try not to fret, as worrying is not good for your baby's development, and the benefits of eating oily fish by far outweigh the risks, say researchers who have studied the effects on mothers and babies.

GOOD FOR YOU AND YOUR BABY

The best source of omega-3 fatty acids, which support the development of your baby's brain, eyes, and nervous system, oily fish also contain vitamins B and D, beta-carotene, magnesium, calcium, and highly digestible protein. A large Danish study found that the babies of mothers who ate the most fish had the best-developed cognitive and motor skills; those who ate the least fish had the least developed skills.

Upping your intake in the third trimester is a good idea: research from Laval University, Quebec, suggests this supports a baby's cognitive, sensory, and motor development, while a study published in the *Journal of Clinical Nutrition* found that babies of mothers who did so slept better. A 2004 study established that eating oily fish boosts birth weight, protecting a baby's health into later life. It also seems to speed post-natal recovery and reduce the risk of the baby blues, mood swings, and depression. Keep eating oily fish as you nurse; omega-3s make breastmilk more brain-nurturing.

The oily properties of the fish are the source of its goodness. But they are part of the problem, too: the oil stores methyl mercury, which fish absorb from polluted waters and their diet of smaller fish. When you eat the fish, this mercury accumulates in your body, taking at least a year to clear out (breastfeeding does this effectively, pumping the toxins into the baby). Mercury is a known teratogen, crossing the placenta and, in large doses, impairing the development of the brain and nervous system. Oily fish can also be contaminated with other pollutants, including dioxins and polychlorinated biphenyls (PCBs). Despite this, the health benefits of eating fish and breastfeeding well outweigh the risks.

To make the most of the good qualities yet safeguard yourself, eat no more than two servings a week (canned tuna doesn't count) of a variety of oily fish from low on the food chain (see below). Do not eat more than two tuna steaks or four medium cans of skipjack tuna a week. It's best to avoid canned "white" or albacore tuna, which may contain higher amounts of mercury.

Avoid raw fish. In some countries, pregnant women are advised to avoid smoked salmon because of risk of listeria.

BUYING NOTES

The freshest place to buy fish is on the harborside as the ice-packed catch is thrown from day-boat to quay. Failing that, support a fish merchant who buys from fishermen and the markets they sell to. You don't have to live near the sea; find one online who will deliver straight to your doorstep.

When buying fish in the supermarket, favor sustainably caught fish: look for those that are individually tagged, marked rod-and-line caught, or sport the Marine Stewardship Council (MSC) logo. Line-caught wild fish are not only better for the environment, safeguarding traditional fishing practices and young fish, they are less flabby than farmed fish. Buy fresh fish that is displayed on ice in a refrigerated cabinet. If buying frozen, gently feel the pack to ensure it is frozen solid, especially if the pack is on the top. Avoid packs that are damaged and covered in ice crystals.

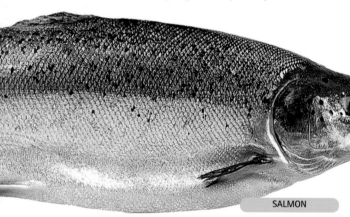

SALMON

Mackerel, herring, trout, sardines, and
salmon are the richest sources
of omega-3 fatty acids

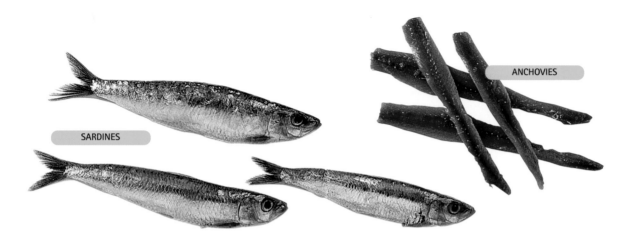

ANCHOVIES

SARDINES

Anchovies, herrings (or pilchards), mackerel, wild salmon (raised without growth promoters and artificial colorants), and organically farmed salmon and trout are not high in pollutants, nor are they overfished. Avoid predator fish high up the food chain, which absorb most mercury, such as swordfish, shark, and marlin.

Fresh fish does not have a fishy smell; just the ozoney whiff of the ocean. The freshest have bright eyes, shiny scales, and pink, feathery edged gills. Press the flesh; it should spring back (just-landed fish is hard to the touch). Fillets and steaks should look fresh and translucent (not milky white).

Canning makes the bones of small fish such as anchovies and sardines more easily digestible. Canning sardines and pilchards does not reduce omega-3 levels, but canning tuna does.

Fish flash-frozen on board the trawler may be fresher than the "fresh" fish in the chiller cabinet.

CULINARY DOS AND DON'TS

- Serve fish the day you buy it.
- Frozen fish that is dry, white or discolored is suffering from freezer burn; don't use.
- Bake fish in foil if you find the smell makes you nauseous.
- Oily fish grills well because it's oily; grill on both sides.
- Check that fish is cooked through; it should be opaque all the way through and the flakes should separate when you stick in a knife.
- It's fine to eat sushi if the fish has been frozen (at -4°F for 24 hours or longer); to be sure of this make it yourself.
- For extra calcium and phosphorus, crunch down the bones of tiny fish and canned salmon.

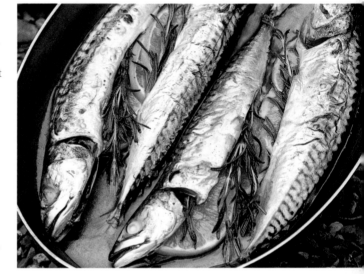

Mackerel (above) is in season all year and tastes best when baked, grilled, or steamed. To counterbalance the richness of the meat, marinate the fish in a vinegar, cider, and spice mix.

QUICK AND EASY DISHES

- *Mash canned sardines on whole-wheat toast, add a few shakes of vinegar, a little black pepper and broil until toasty.*
- *Add salmon to scrambled eggs with a bit of cream for a special breakfast or brunch. Serve it on whole-wheat toast with a sprinkling of black pepper.*

oily fish

SEAFOOD

Eating seafood is a tasty way to take in essential nutrients during pregnancy, when large amounts of food can make you feel uncomfortably full. Make sure seafood has been thoroughly cooked or frozen (which kills bacteria and parasites such as tapeworm). During pregnancy the immune system is suppressed, making you more susceptible to food poisoning.

GOOD FOR YOU AND YOUR BABY
Shellfish of all types is a fabulous source of calcium, iodine, selenium, iron, zinc, and protein, as well as one of the best sources of omega-3 fatty acids. However, studies suggest that crab may have the same levels of pollutants, including dioxins and PCBs, as oily fish (see page 56), so don't eat more than two portions of brown crabmeat a week.

Raw seafood harbors bacteria including salmonella; clams, oysters, and mussels from polluted waters pose the greatest risk of food poisoning, but cooking to more than 145°F destroys the bacteria.

HARVESTING NOTES
To be extra safe during pregnancy, buy from a trusted supplier. Langoustine and shrimp, squid and octopus, clams, mussels, oysters, and scallops are all good pregnancy meal choices.

Buy bivalves alive for safety as much as for taste. A fish merchant is more likely to have live seafood than a supermarket, or look for date-stamped deliveries of live items brought direct to your door less than 24 hours after harvesting. Commercially farmed bivalves should have been treated with ultraviolet light to make them safe. When buying from markets, ask where the seafood came from, and whether the waters were certified clean.

Choose fresh dived scallops over those already opened and dressed, and creel-caught langoustines. Shrimp from the North Atlantic are said to have the best taste. Select clams, mussels, and oysters with closed shells; if they don't close when you tap them sharply, discard. Serve the day you buy. Freezing squid, however, maintains the

---

Shrimp are a low-fat source of protein
and are high in potassium and zinc.
They also contain omega-3 fatty acids.

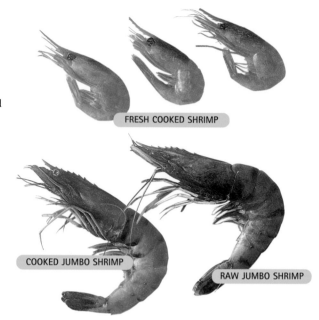

FRESH COOKED SHRIMP

COOKED JUMBO SHRIMP

RAW JUMBO SHRIMP

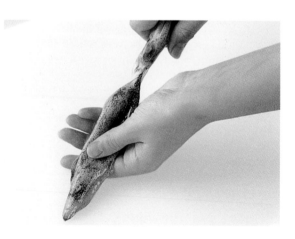

When preparing squid, make sure you remove the head, the bony support inside the pouch, and the transparent membrane that covers the body. The pouch, tentacles, fins, and ink are all edible; the ink can even be used to give flavor and color to risotto and pasta.

nutrients and can make the fibers less tough. When choosing frozen shrimp, choose uncooked ones still in their shells. Fresh ones should have perky eyes and glossy, nicely colored shells. Never leave frozen or defrosted shrimp lying around in a warm room, as the natural bacteria they contain will cause them to spoil very rapidly and possibly cause poisoning.

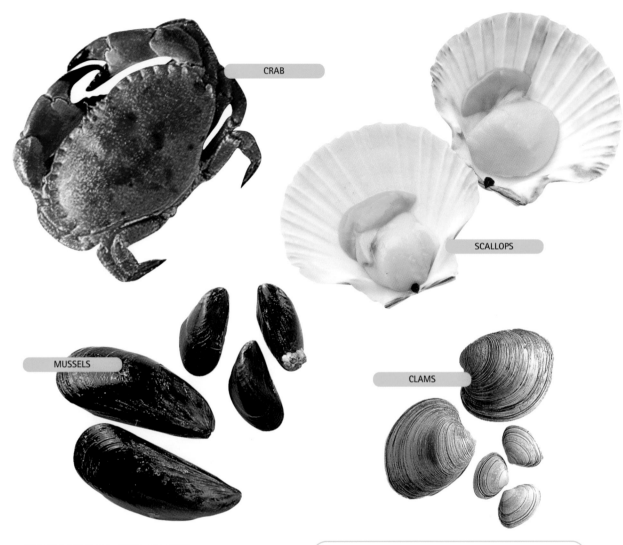

CRAB

SCALLOPS

MUSSELS

CLAMS

CULINARY DOS AND DON'TS

- Don't eat bivalves raw during pregnancy.
- Always cook seafood thoroughly. Whether boiled, grilled, or stir-fried, raw shrimp should turn pink.
- If the shells of clams, mussels, and oysters remain shut after cooking, discard them.
- Pull away the hair-like strands attached to the hinge of mussel shells. Rinse in cold water and scrub with a small, hard-bristled brush.
- Soak cleaned mussels and clams in a bowl of lightly salted cold water for 2–3 hours, changing the water if it muddies. A handful of oats in the water may help the shellfish disgorge any grit.
- Add clams to pasta dishes dressed with oil and garlic.
- For tender squid, either cook very quickly over high heat (for 2–3 minutes) or braise slowly (for more than 30 minutes).

QUICK AND EASY DISHES

- *Steam mussels in white wine with a little garlic and some finely chopped shallots (the alcohol is lost in the cooking). Stir in sour cream just before serving. Accompany with crusty bread.*
- *Cook jumbo shrimp and serve with sweet chili sauce and sesame seed dip. Accompany with tender asparagus spears and a whisked mustard, vinegar, and brown sugar sauce.*
- *Serve freshly cooked shelled shrimp over a bed of shredded lettuce with a spicy tomato sauce.*

seafood

SEAWEED

This traditional fertility tonic has been valued by generations of Japanese mothers, who swear that eating seaweed produces a baby with a full head of lustrous hair. Seaweed absorbs a rich blend of vitamins and minerals from the sea, including the iodine required for a healthy thyroid gland, which has to work harder during pregnancy. Herbalists may recommend seaweed during pregnancy to aid digestion and counter constipation, to cleanse and strengthen circulation, lift depression and energy levels, and counter aches and anemia. If you pick your own, you can look forward to relaxing seashore walks, too.

Look for dried Japanese seaweeds in health food stores. Rehydrate following packet instructions. Capsules are neither as nutritionally effective nor as tasty as the dried or fresh vegetable.

Sheets of black nori (laver) are best for wrapping sushi, while for soups kombu (kelp) adds a tangy taste, and dark green wakame (kelp) is milder and requires less cooking. Sweet arame (kelp) suits vegetable stir-fries, while agar (carragheen) is used as a setting agent.

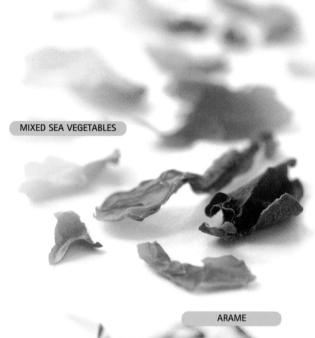

MIXED SEA VEGETABLES

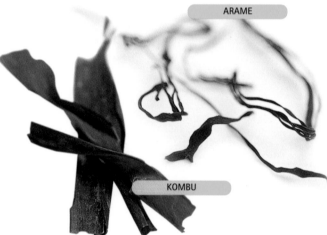

ARAME

KOMBU

GLOSSY HAIR RINSE

Seaweed is an age-old recipe for lustrous locks. Researchers at the University of Leeds have found that seaweed has evolved to protect itself from "weathering" and can help your hair withstand the elements, too.

2 strips of kombu, nori, or arame

1 Soak the strips of seaweed in boiling water for 30 minutes. Hook out with a slotted spoon to use in cooking, reserving the water.
2 Wash and condition your hair as usual. Towel dry, then apply the reserved seaweed water to your damp hair. Wrap hair in a plastic bag and a warm towel, then relax for 30 minutes.
3 Rinse your hair with plenty of warm, then gradually cooler water.
4 Finally, dry and style your hair as you would normally.

GOOD FOR YOU AND YOUR BABY

One of the most vitamin- and mineral-rich plants there is, containing beta-carotene, vitamins C, E, K, folate, and many B vitamins—seaweed is one of the best sources of B_{12}. It contains some 23 minerals, too, among them iodine, calcium, selenium, magnesium, zinc, copper, and manganese, plus fluorine for healthy teeth and bones. Seaweed is fiber filled and an important vegetable protein for those who don't eat meat. It also supplies omega-3 fatty acids. Seaweed's blend of phytonutrients is strongly antioxidant, containing polysaccharides and peptides that aid the immune system and alignic acid, considered useful for ridding the body of heavy metals and other seaborne pollutants. Herbalists think of seaweed as a cleansing and immune-supporting plant, and it is also used as a tonic for the skin and hair. If you are watching your salt intake, be aware that seaweed has a high sodium content. Avoid hijiki, which may contain arsenic, and all seaweed if you are allergic to iodine. Kelp and wracks can be very high in iodine, so check with your doctor if this might be a problem.

HARVESTING NOTES

The best sources are away-from-it-all bays in unpolluted waters. Avoid seaweed growing near heavy industry or nuclear plants. When picking your own, investigate the water quality by talking to your water authority or environment agency. Also find out whether the coastline is owned, and whether you need permission before collecting seaweed.

Spring and early summer are the best times to pick new fronds. Collect them as the tide is going out. Laver is traditionally collected in the fall. Take a good identification guide with you (some seaweeds aren't as tasty as others, some might cause stomach pains and others are rare or protected). Make sure the weed is alive and rooted to rocks before you cut (above the top of the stem so part of the frond is still attached to the rock), and harvest only a little from each site. Newly washed up dead weed makes a good garden mulch and fertilizer.

CULINARY DOS AND DON'TS

- Never eat seaweed raw from the sea.
- Rinse fresh seaweed in several changes of water to remove salt and grit.
- Dry washed seaweed in a very low oven until dark brown and crumbly. Store in an airtight container.
- Soak dried seaweed for 30 minutes before adding to soups and stir-fries.
- Sprinkle dried seaweed over salads and rice dishes or use as a seasoning.
- Toast nori before using. Place over a flame for a few seconds (holding with tongs), or place on a baking sheet and put in a hot oven for 30–60 seconds.
- Deep-fry crispy sea lettuce to eat as a snack.
- Dulse is delicious served in salads, soups, stews, or blanched vegetable dishes.
- Add wakame to soups or salads.
- Try oaty-tasting laver bread, made from Welsh purple laver.
- Cooking legumes with kombu shortens cooking time. Just place some of the seaweed in a pan with beans or peas and water and cook as normal.

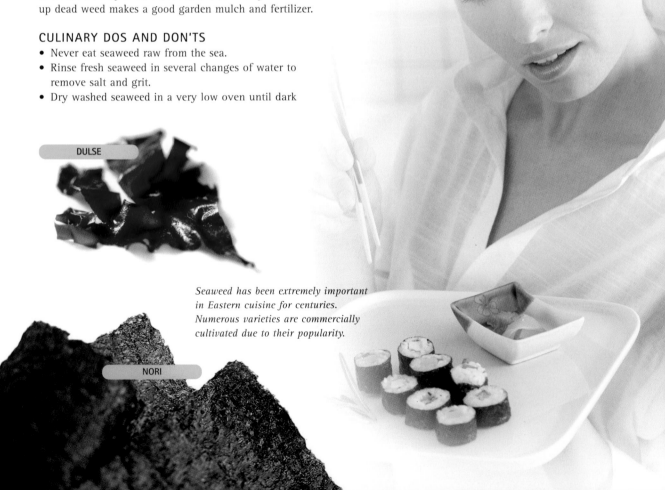

DULSE

NORI

Seaweed has been extremely important in Eastern cuisine for centuries. Numerous varieties are commercially cultivated due to their popularity.

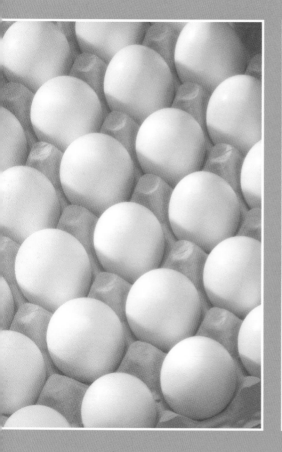
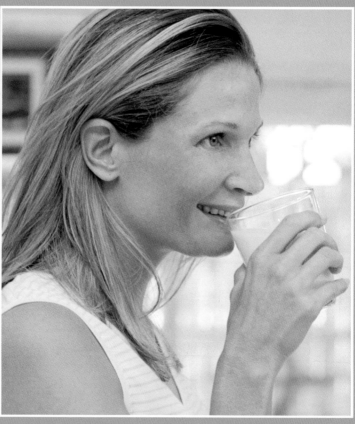
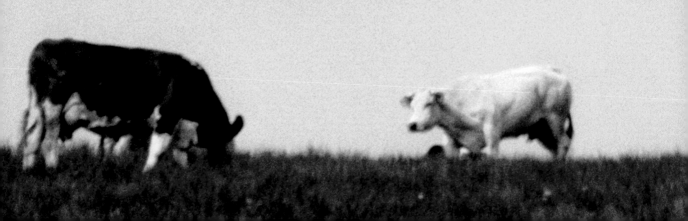

GREAT EATING FROM THE FARM

The healthiest and most ethical meat and dairy products come from animals raised outdoors, where they can absorb the goodness of the sun and grass, and behave as Mother Nature intended. Animals that forage on grass have two to four times more omega-3 fatty acids—these build your baby's brain and nervous system—than those reared intensively indoors on an unnatural diet based on grain or soy. Suppliers of organic meat should be able to tell you from which supplier their food comes.

POULTRY • RABBIT • MEAT • EGGS
YOGURT • CHEESE • MILK

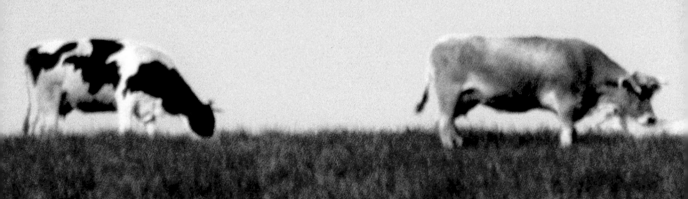

POULTRY

Chicken is one of the most comforting ways to obtain the extra B vitamins, minerals, and protein you need during pregnancy. When you feel in need of cosseting, try roasting a chicken or making chicken soup. For a treat, why not try a goose, which is even higher in protein? Look for organic, free range or traditional eating breeds to ensure the best quality meat and to reassure yourself that the bird enjoyed a good life.

GOOD FOR YOU AND YOUR BABY

Packed with B vitamins, iron, zinc, selenium, and phosphorus, poultry is one of the most easily absorbed sources of protein. Make sure you eat some brown meat, which is higher in minerals. Chicken and turkey are generally lower in fat than red meat. Removing the skin lowers the saturated fat content more, but reduces taste and succulence, since flavor and moistness are carried in fat molecules. Factory-farmed chickens are more fatty than those reared organically—researchers at London Metropolitan University found that the average factory-farmed chicken has more fat than protein thanks to its breeding for size, lack of exercise, and diet. Since 1980, changes in diet have seen a dramatic reduction in omega-3 fatty acids in chicken, too. Organic chicken contains more protein.

Geese, often thought of as fatty, are far lower in fat than beef or lamb, and contain more protein than chicken or turkey. They graze on grass, which produces a wild, red meat-like flavor. Goose fat is a good cooking medium, and one of the most healthy animal fats, containing fewer saturated fats and more mono-and polyunsaturated fats than butter or lard.

RABBIT

Rabbit is often described as having the flavor of an old-fashioned chicken, and makes a useful alternative. It is as low-fat as chicken but contains more iron.

BUYING NOTES

Buy organic or free range, which supports lower density stocking and allows birds the freedom to roam and act like chickens (rather than meat machines). The words "slow-grown," "organic," "traditional free range," or "unlimited area" denote that the bird has ventured outdoors. "Free range" may not mean as free or able to roam as it suggests, nor that stocking density permits normal bird behavior. Favor systems in which chickens spend the day outdoors—"visit" the farm online to find out more. Heritage breeds are always mentioned on the pack (and command a higher price).

Choose chickens reared for longer than the eight-week intensive cycle; 20 weeks or more allows time for flavor and nutrients to develop.

Corn-fed birds have a better flavor—chickens traditionally eat corn, not soy or fishmeal. Organic standards are the most rigorous on stocking density and the birds' diet.

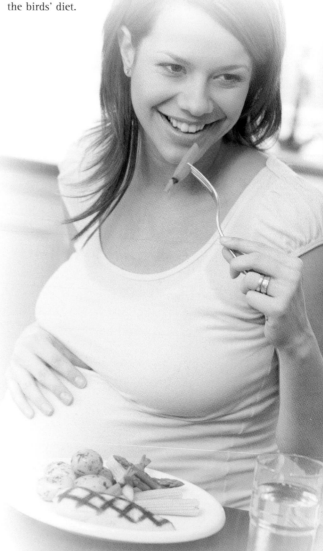

Skinless chicken that is broiled or baked and served with a mix of steamed vegetables provides a healthy meal that is high in protein and vitamins.

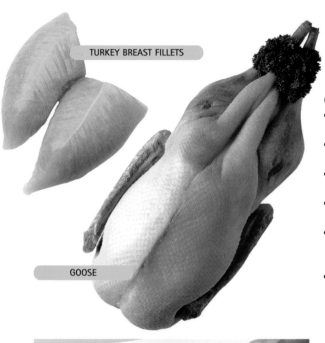

TURKEY BREAST FILLETS

GOOSE

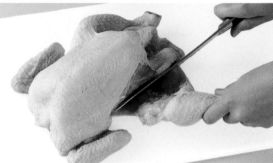

come from unregulated sources that allow adulteration. Check the small print for sodium; unadulterated chicken is 100 percent chicken.

CULINARY DOS AND DON'TS

- To spot an intensively reared chicken, look for signs of ammonia burns on the knee joints.
- Store raw poultry in a refrigerator in a container so the juices don't touch other food.
- Keep a separate cutting board for preparing raw meat and clean well after use.
- Wash your hands and any implements used well after handling all raw poultry .
- Cook poultry until the juices run clear when you stick in a knife; if they are pink, the bird needs more cooking. Alternatively, use a cooking thermometer.
- Prick goose skin before roasting to allow the fat to run off. Then set it on a trivet or rack inside a roasting pan to catch the fat, or transfer to another pan halfway through cooking; reserve the fat for roasting potatoes.
- Use leftover cold roast chicken in salads and sandwiches.
- Don't discard the carcass; make a stock (see page 118) to raise the nutritional profile and taste of soups and rice dishes.

The widest choice of turkeys—organic and free range—is usually available at Thanksgiving, but parts are available all year round.

Geese cannot be farmed intensively, so you are assured of a free-ranging bird. If you already keep chickens for eggs, you might try raising broiler chicks (this means raising male chicks separately). Slower growing, traditional breeds have more flavor.

In the United States, poultry carcasses are routinely washed in chlorine to kill bacteria; they are banned in the EU, as chlorine has not been proven safe to ingest.

Avoid processed chicken products—pies, curries, stir-fries – which contain high levels of fat and additives. Some supermarket chicken has been "enhanced"—injected with "chicken broth" or salt water and additives such as proteins. This is even more likely with chicken used in processed foods or served in canteens and restaurants, which is almost always reared intensively, on high-protein, antibiotic-laced feed. The meat may

QUICK AND EASY DISHES

- *Stir-fry strips of chicken in a little walnut oil with chopped red bell pepper, scallion and broccoli florets. Add a dash of soy sauce and roll up in a warm pancake.*
- *Joint a whole chicken and add to a soupy stew of onion, garlic, ginger, tomato, and spices. Allow to cook slowly for an hour, then stir in yogurt just before serving.*
- *Sauté chicken pieces, then add a little white wine, tomatoes, and soaked dried porcini mushrooms with their soaking water; simmer over low heat until cooked through and serve with polenta.*
- *Marinate chicken or turkey breast overnight in yogurt with garlic, onion, sweet paprika, and a little mint, then thread onto skewers and broil; serve with a watercress salad.*

poultry

MEAT

Red meat is so nutrient-dense that you don't need huge portions to ensure good nutrition—useful when your stomach is squashed by a growing baby. Since, however, you deserve the best in pregnancy, so, too, do the animals that provide you with those much-needed nutrients. You can ensure both by choosing livestock reared on pasture, which contains the natural goodness of grass and all the flavor of Mother Earth. Animals that eat grass rather than processed feed produce meat lower in saturated fat and higher in omega-3 fatty acids; the meat has a better texture and flavor, too. Indeed, when cattle are pastured on grass, their meat is almost as lean as wild game.

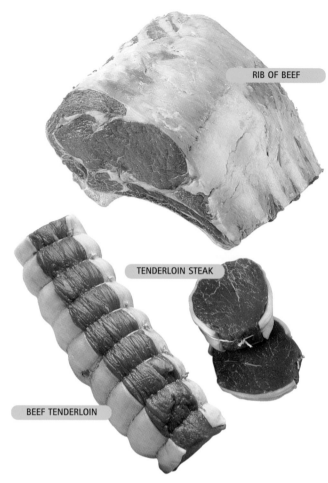

RIB OF BEEF

TENDERLOIN STEAK

BEEF TENDERLOIN

GOOD FOR YOU AND YOUR BABY

Red meat, such as beef and lamb, is the best and most easily absorbed natural source of iron and zinc, B vitamins, and protein. Beef is more nutrient-rich than lamb, which has the most fat of any red meat. Venison is lower in fat than beef, lamb, and even chicken, and is high in polyunsaturates. Avoid liver during pregnancy, which is too high in vitamin A to be safe.

Pregnancy makes you more susceptible to food poisoning and stomach bugs, so avoid raw meat and "rare" cooking methods, which raise the risk of salmonella poisoning and infection with the parasite toxoplasmosis. The latter can damage a developing baby's brain and eyes. Avoid pâtés if they have not been pasteurized or UHT treated to kill the listeria bug. In some countries, cured meat such as ham or salume is contraindicated during pregnancy because of the listeria risk. This advice is not given in the UK. US stock may have been treated with additives such as steroids and growth hormones to produce leaner meat; this practice is outlawed in the EU.

BUYING NOTES

Buy meat direct from farmers who practice good husbandry when you can. What's the best way to research this? Visit the farm online, or chat with your butcher or the farmer at farmers' markets. Organic

standards are the most stringent on stocking density, time spent outdoors, and feed. If you do go out into the country, avoid close contact with sheep during lambing season. The animals may harbour chlamydiosis, toxoplasmosis, and listeriosis, which carry a risk of infection and miscarriage.

Favor farmers who graze their stock on grass, which is richer in vitamins E and beta-carotene than hay or grain. Animals that graze on pasture have higher levels of omega-3 than those fed grain and soy. Grazing cattle also supply more B vitamins, calcium, magnesium, and potassium—and less fat. The joy of lamb is that animals are free to roam on grass, though "new season" lamb for Easter may be more intensively reared. Good husbandry costs, so the best-raised meat is not always the cheapest. To get more for your money (and put more in the farmer's pocket) cut out middlemen by buying direct from farm stores and farmers' markets. Many will deliver to your door.

Taste tests show that grass-fed meat (pasture in summer; hay or silage in winter) has greatest flavor. Ask your butcher or the farmer how the meat is hung, and

---

In Nepal, a craving for meat in pregnancy is
said to betoken a boy.

---

how this affects the taste and texture. When choosing red meat, look for marbling (lines of fat); this shows the animal was well cared for and grew to maturity slowly and outdoors. Traditional butchers don't package meat in plastic because they know it has to breathe. Select firm-textured meat that looks shiny not wet, and holds the dent if you press your thumb into it.

If you're worried about saturated fat, don't cut out meat itself, just processed meat—burgers, pies, ready meals—which tends to be higher in fat and additives, and may contain MRM, mechanically recovered meat. Deli meats aren't a good idea: you don't know how long they've been stored and at what temperature; they may harbour the listeria bug.

Hotdogs and sausages may contain nitrates, so are best avoided. Organic sausages and prepared meat products contain fewer additives. In the United States, ask for hormone-free meat.

CULINARY DOS AND DON'TS

- Store raw meat in a container in the refrigerator so the juices don't touch other food.
- Keep a separate cutting board for raw meat and clean well after use.
- Wash your hands and any implements used after handling raw meat.
- Ask for steaks well done when eating out, no matter your preference before pregnancy.
- Broil rather than fry in fat to reduce the total fat content. To retain flavor and succulence, cut off the fat after cooking rather than before
- Brown pieces of meat in a little oil to seal in flavor before casseroling.
- Beef consommé is a traditional postpartum soup to rebuild strength.

QUICK AND EASY DISHES

- *Stir-fry cubes of beef with chopped onion, ginger, star anise, black pepper, and soy sauce; throw in broccoli florets at the end.*
- *For a quick stew, brown cubes of beef, add to a casserole with halved onion, cubed rutabaga and celeriac, roughly chopped parsnips and carrots, quartered potatoes, and vegetable stock. Cook over low heat for at least 1 hour, adding sliced cabbage just before serving.*
- *Brown cubes of lamb; in another pan fry red onion with garlic, cubed eggplant, and a few cumin seeds, add a little water and steam until gloopy. Combine the lamb and eggplant with yogurt, and if you can take the heat, serve with harissa.*
- *Fry onions, garlic, and ginger with a few cloves, add some ground lamb and a little turmeric, a couple of plum tomatoes, and diced potatoes, then simmer until the potatoes are just done.*

- Sounds strange, but anchovies bring out something in lamb. Also try studding a lamb joint with garlic and rosemary before roasting.
- Middle Eastern flavors, such as pomegranate, eggplant, yogurt, and preserved lemon, marry well with lamb.
- Venison's traditional accompaniments are red or black currants and it goes well with caramelized parsnips.
- Try substituting venison where you would use beef.

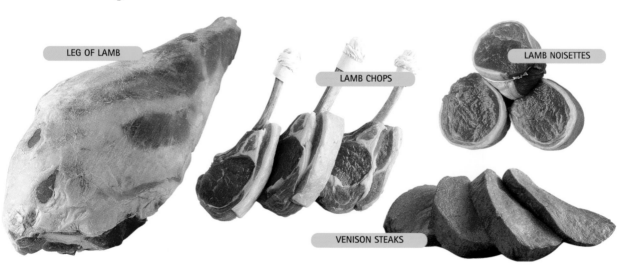

LEG OF LAMB

LAMB CHOPS

LAMB NOISETTES

VENISON STEAKS

EGGS

A symbol of new life and potential, and of mother and baby in cultures around the globe, eggs are without doubt one of the best foods for nurturing new life. It's traditional in Jewish households to give a new baby an egg. Start your day with them; a study from the University of Massachusetts found that eating eggs for breakfast kept people feeling 50 percent more sated than breakfast cereals did.

GOOD FOR YOU AND YOUR BABY

Within the shell of an egg is contained everything necessary to grow a chick, so it's no wonder these are such a fabulous food source for expectant mothers. Inside the shell lie vitamins B_2, B_5, B_{12} and D, selenium, iodine, phosphorus, and choline, without which you can become deficient in folate (do eat the yolk, where the choline is). The UN has pronounced the egg a better source of protein than milk, fish, beef, and legumes. Eggs also contain more of the carotenoids lutein and zeaxanthin—antioxidants vital for eye health—than spinach. Duck eggs have more protein than hen's eggs.

During pregnancy, avoid raw and soft-cooked eggs to reduce the risk of salmonella bacteria. This means no homemade mayonnaise or meringues (bought versions are usually okay; check they are pasteurized). Although it is unlikely to harm your baby, salmonella can make you very ill, and during pregnancy the immune system is not as vigilant as usual.

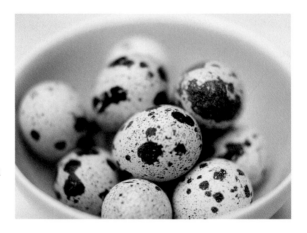

BUYING NOTES

Favor eggs from birds raised on grass: they can contain almost ten times as many omega-3 fatty acids and up to six times more vitamin E then eggs from indoor hens. A 2007 study found that grass-raised eggs have a third less cholesterol and a quarter less saturated fat, but two-thirds more vitamin A than indoor eggs.

Egg boxes labeled "free range" and even "organic" aren't an assurance that hens have been raised on pasture. You're more likely to source nutritionally rich outdoor eggs at farmers' markets, farm stores and from people who keep a few chooks.
Reject boxes with cracked eggs and eggs past their sell-by date. Store eggs separately from other food.

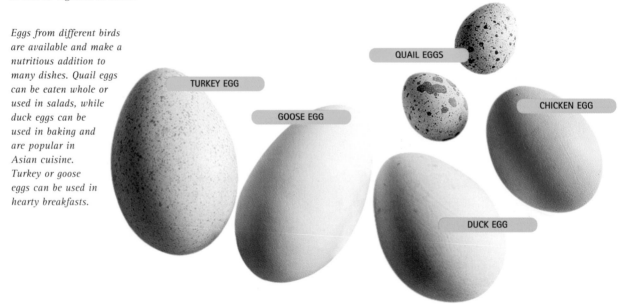

Eggs from different birds are available and make a nutritious addition to many dishes. Quail eggs can be eaten whole or used in salads, while duck eggs can be used in baking and are popular in Asian cuisine. Turkey or goose eggs can be used in hearty breakfasts.

TURKEY EGG

GOOSE EGG

QUAIL EGGS

CHICKEN EGG

DUCK EGG

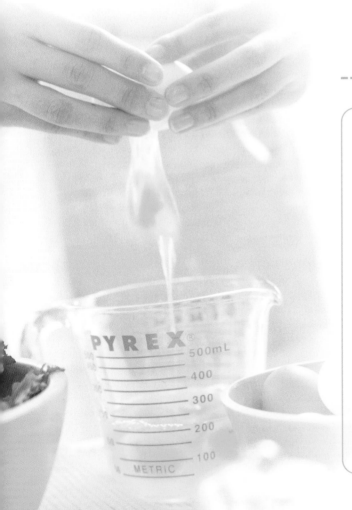

CULINARY DOS AND DON'TS

- To check an egg for freshness, place it in water; the older it is, the more likely it is to float (eggs lose water and gain air during storage).
- Wash your hands, cooking equipment, and surfaces after cracking or handling eggs in their shell.
- Boil eggs for seven minutes or longer to kill salmonella bacteria.
- During pregnancy poach eggs until the white is completely white and the yolk is hard.
- Flip fried eggs to cook on both sides, for safety.
- If eggs aren't your morning favorite, disguise them in a pancake batter, or eat egg-based breads such as panettone and challah.

During pregnancy avoid raw and soft-cooked eggs to reduce the risk of ingesting salmonella bacteria.

QUICK AND EASY DISHES

- *For a quick breakfast, try French toast. Soak slices of bread in eggs beaten with a pinch of salt, then gently fry in a little butter. Serve with a sprinkling of cinnamon or a little maple syrup.*
- *When scrambling eggs, stir in strips of smoked salmon to heat through before serving with plenty of black pepper and shavings of Parmesan.*
- *Gently fry sliced garlic, red bell pepper, and ripe tomatoes in olive oil until soft and fragrant, then add sliced scallion and beaten eggs and stir. When set, serve with slices of crusty bread*
- *For an easy dessert, beat 2 whole eggs and 2 yolks with 2 tbsp sugar, 2 cups whole milk, and 1 tsp vanilla extract. Pour into ramekins standing in a baking dish of hot water, cover with foil making a hole in the center, and bake in a low oven for 2 hours, until set. Chill before serving with toasted almond slices.*

eggs

MILK, YOGURT, AND CHEESE

The image of cows with their calves is a byword for motherhood across the globe, and milk in some form is a daily necessity during pregnancy for healthy bones and teeth. Cheese concentrates the goodness of milk into nutrient-rich parcels—you only need a little to get your daily fill of calcium and protein—and yogurt has so many health benefits it is cited as a causal factor in longevity in communities around the world. Dairy produce is considered so nurturing to the life-force in India that a new mother is given a combination of milk, clarified butter, and honey to rebuild her strength.

GOOD FOR YOU AND YOUR BABY

Milk is a fantastic source of calcium and vitamins D and K—a combination that supports bone health. It also contains beta-carotene and B vitamins, iodine and potassium and omega-3 fatty acids. It's a high protein food. A 1999 study found that the milk of cows raised on grass is richest in vitamins. Whole milk contains the most beta-carotene and conjugated linoleic acid (CLA), but also more saturated fat.

Yogurt shares the vitamin and mineral load of milk, but supplies more calcium. Its live bacteria— *Lactobacillus bulgaricus* or *acidophilus*, *Streptococcus thermophilus* or *Bifidobacteria*—produce not only the distinctive sour taste, but enhance immunity and speed recovery from infection. If you are prone to yeast infection in pregnancy, eat 6 tbsp live yogurt daily (in one study this reduced the incidence of infection threefold). Yogurt also lessens inflammation in IBS flare-ups, and seems effective against bad breath, a problem in pregnancy when you can't breathe comfortably through your nose or have gum problems. Eating 6 tbsp sugar-free yogurt twice daily for six weeks reduced symptoms in one study. Research into probiotics in pregnancy has linked yogurt with the prevention of atopic eczema in babies. Using yogurt with live active cultures vaginally also seems to reduce the risk of developing infections that can lead to premature labor.

A University of Aberdeen study found organic cheese to be higher in omega-3 fatty acids than organic milk. During pregnancy it's safest to eat cheese made from pasteurized rather than "raw" milk (check the label), and to avoid soft, mold-ripened cheeses—Brie or Camembert, goat cheeses with a white rind—and blue cheeses Stilton, Dolcelatte, and Gorgonzola. Bacteria that is harmful during pregnancy, such as listeria, are more likely to grow on these cheeses. Cooking kills these cheese bacteria. Softer cheeses that are safe to eat include feta, ricotta, mascarpone, and mozzarella.

BUYING NOTES

Choose organic products from cows reared on pasture for the best taste, maximum nutrients, and peace of mind about animal ethics. Organic milk will reduce your exposure to fat-soluble toxins such as pesticides. A University of Aberdeen study found that organic milk contained up to 71 percent higher amounts of omega-3 fatty acids than conventional milk. The researchers put the benefits down to red clover in the pastures (a traditional pregnancy tonic herb). Small local dairies are more likely to offer milk from cows grazed on pasture.

Research from 1998 found double the amount of CLA in French than American cheeses, and put this down to the habit of rearing cows on pasture. Pastured dairies the world over produce milk with similar advantages.

Check the label before buying your milk. Different types of milk contain varying amounts of calories, protein, fat, and vitamins A and B complex.

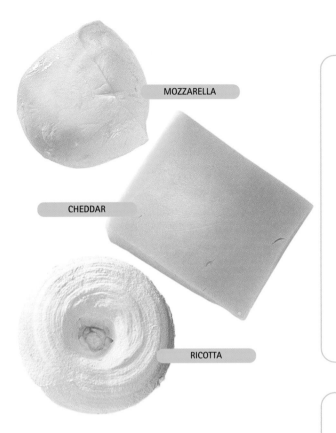

MOZZARELLA

CHEDDAR

RICOTTA

QUICK AND EASY DISHES

- *Add 1 tbsp honey to a bowl of yogurt and sprinkle with toasted sunflower and pumpkin seeds.*
- *As an accompaniment to grilled meat, serve yogurt mixed with chopped cucumber, dried mint, lemon juice, and black pepper.*
- *Top a baked potato with thick yogurt, chives, and black pepper.*
- *For instant pizza, spread very ripe tomatoes onto French bread, add a sprinkling of dried Herbes de Provence and sliced mozzarella, then broil until bubbling.*
- *Cut feta into cubes, dust with oregano and combine with ripe tomatoes, chunks of cucumber, and black olives.*

Choose yogurt labeled "live" to be sure that it contains the fermenting bacteria that confer so many health benefits. Fruit-flavored yogurt will be high in sugar and often includes additives and thickening agents. It's always healthier to buy plain yogurt with live active cultures and add your own fresh fruit.

If you cannot tolerate cow's milk, substitute goat or sheep's milk and their yogurt or cheeses, which are often tolerated better.

CULINARY DOS AND DON'TS

- Ditch additive-filled chocolate drinks; instead heat a mug of milk, add 1–2 tsp unsweetened cocoa powder and a spoonful of honey. Stir well to mix.
- Add low-fat yogurt to muesli and granola.
- Substitute rich Greek yogurt where cream is called for to top desserts.
- Cool spicy curries and other chili-hot dishes with a side helping of yogurt.
- Freeze yogurt as an alternative to ice cream.

BANANA SMOOTHIE

For a healthy start to the day, make this delicious smoothie for an energy-rich breakfast.

1 ripe banana, peeled and sliced
1¼ cups milk
1 handful of ice
1–2 tbsp pasteurized honey

Place the banana, milk, ice, and honey in a blender and blend until smooth. Transfer to a drinking glass and serve at once.

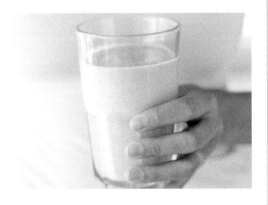

milk, yogurt, and cheese

MAKING YOGURT AT HOME

If you make your own yogurt you can be sure of the provenance of the ingredients, keeping them organic and ethically sourced. Once you have made your first batch, within a week use 2–3 tbsp as a starter for the new batch. Make sure that your equipment, worktop, and hands are scrupulously clean before you start. You can buy yogurt starter mix at health food stores.

You will need:

4 cups whole milk
¼ cup powdered milk
2–3 tbsp yogurt with live active cultures or 1 envelope yogurt starter (unflavored and unsweetened)
6–8 (⅔ cup) glass jars with airtight lids or plastic wrap

1 First sterilize all the equipment (cooking thermometer, thick-bottomed metal pan with a lid, metal spoon, measuring cup, glass jars and lids, if using, by running them through the hottest cycle in a dishwasher or wash well with detergent in hot water, then dry in a low oven.

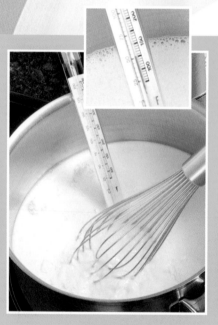
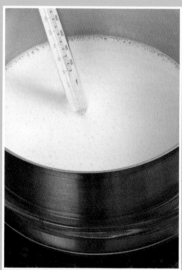
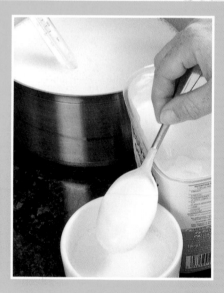

2 Heat the fresh and powdered milk in a heavy metal saucepan to 185-195°F and maintain it at this temperature, stirring, without allowing it to boil for 10 minutes. This sterilizes the milk and kills bacteria.

3 Now cool the milk rapidly by plunging the pan into a large bowl of ice or cold water (don't let the water come over the side into the milk). Allow the pan to sit until the temperature has dropped to 122°F.

4 Remove the pan from the water and lift out 1 cup of milk. Stir in the live yogurt. Then stir the mixture in the cup into the milk in the pan, distributing it well. Divide the mixture between the sterilized jars, and immediately lid them or wrap tightly in plastic wrap.

Once the yogurt has thickened and set, allow it to cool then refrigerate. It should keep up to 10 days. If you desire, stir in fruit, jelly or pasteurized honey to sweeten just before eating.

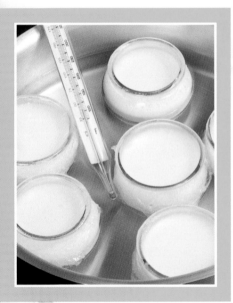

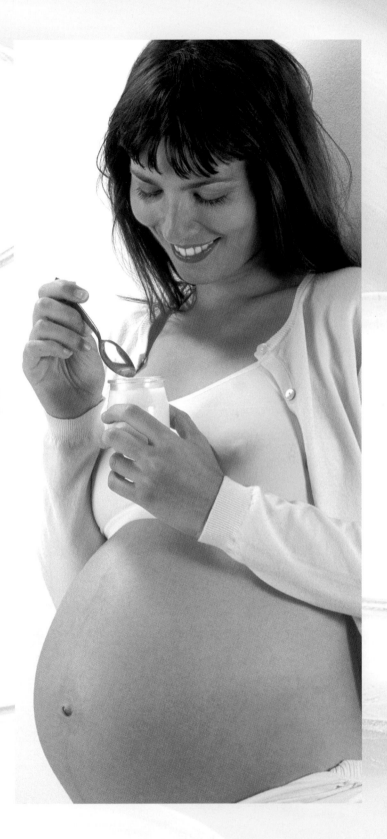

5 Stand the jars in a pan of water heated to 122°F over low heat for 5–6 hours. Don't let the water come over the lids or plastic-wrapped tops. Check the temperature regularly (bacteria won't grow well below 98°F and are killed over 130°F). Top up the water as necessary.

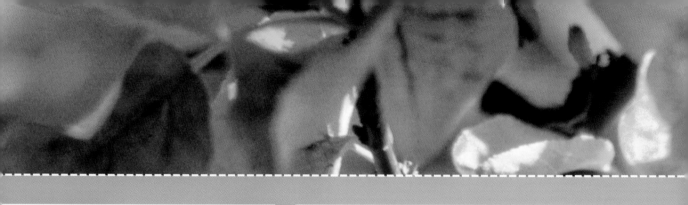
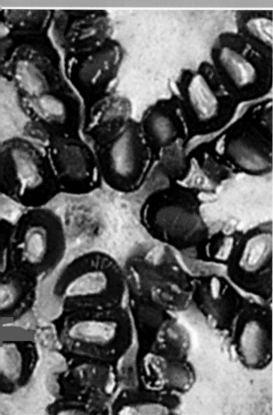
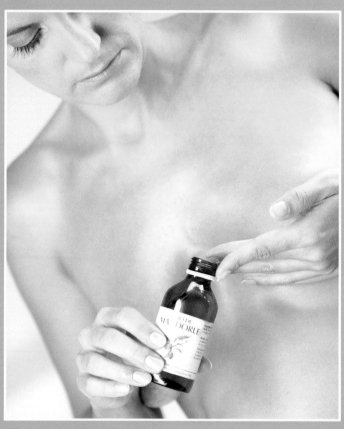
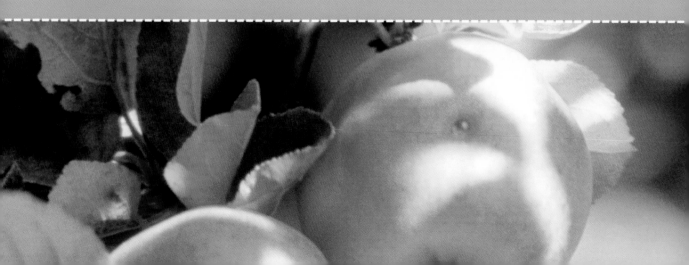

BOUNTY FROM THE ORCHARD

Fruit and nuts make perfect snack food, meeting your increased daily need for nutrients, fiber, and a quick energy boost. Planting your own trees—some can thrive in pots and on balconies—allows you to choose heritage varieties not available in supermarkets for their taste, growing habit, or name associations. It's traditional to plant an apple tree for a boy and a pear tree for a girl.

APPLES • APRICOTS • POMEGRANATES • FIGS
WALNUTS • ALMONDS • AVOCADOS • OLIVES

APPLES

The humble apple is one of the best fruits for health as well as for taste. From Italy to Bulgaria, the apple is linked with conception and the miraculous pregnancies of the Virgin Mary and her mother, Saint Anne.

GOOD FOR YOU AND YOUR BABY

A good source of vitamin C, potassium, and fiber, apples are packed with antioxidant phytonutrients, including the valuable flavonoids quercetin, catechin, and phloridzin, which gather in and around the skin. Quercetin is anti-inflammatory, stops blood from clumping, and regulates blood pressure; catechin is also heart-healthy, while phloridzin offers protection for the lungs if you are prone to asthma. Researchers in the Netherlands and Scotland found that mothers who ate apples in pregnancy significantly reduced their children's risk of developing asthma and wheezing. Pectin in apples is thought to lower blood cholesterol.

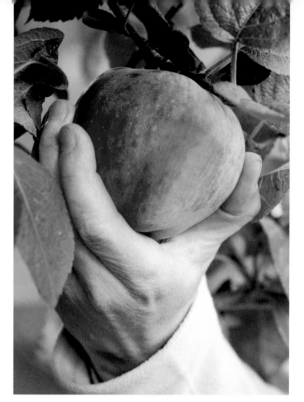

BUYING NOTES

It's just about possible to eat apples year round: the earliest are ready in midsummer and late-ripening fruit are sold until the end of spring. Storing apples does not seem to reduce their phytonutrient levels. Indeed, in one study, apples kept for 200 days were almost as high in flavonoids as when they were harvested.

Since it's nutritionally important to eat the skin, make sure you buy organic. Non-organic apples may be coated with a protective wax made of petroleum, and

the fruit is among the most pesticide-contaminated produce. Wash apples before eating.

Apples in supermarkets can be mealy or tasteless; many are picked unripe from varieties bred not for taste but for ease of transportation. You'll find a far greater choice of apples at local and farmers' markets or pick-your-own farms. Make sure you pick ripe apples: Austrian research has suggested that antioxidant levels rise as fruit ripens.

Look out for Apple Day celebrations and harvest fairs where you can sample and learn about different varieties, from spicy russets to tongue-tingling crispy cooking apples. Favor cloudy apple juice; the pulp protects the cardiovascular system.

CULINARY DOS AND DON'TS

- For baking, choose apples with a creamy texture and sharp flavor.
- Juicing reduces the fruit's antioxidants; after juicing, only 3–10 percent may remain, so do eat whole apples.
- Stewing causes up to 70 percent of flavonols to leach into the cooking water; make sure you use it!
- Keep an apple in your bag: it provides 15 percent of your daily fiber.
- Shred apple into muesli, the traditional Swiss way.

QUICK AND EASY DISHES

- *Core an apple and fill the hole with a mixture of raisins, walnuts, brown sugar, and cinnamon, then bake in a moderate oven until soft.*
- *For a mincemeat filling, dice apples and combine in a jar with raisins, dates, cloves, cinnamon, and suet; moisten with brandy and store in a cool dark place for three months to use in pies.*
- *Make applesauce by stewing dessert apples in a tiny amount of water for 10 minutes. You may not need sugar.*

APRICOTS

Fresh or dried apricots supply plenty of nutrients useful in pregnancy, including vitamin C and potassium. Apricots are considered a folk treatment for infertility and the oil is a standard base for stretch-mark lotions.

GOOD FOR YOU AND YOUR BABY

A delicious source of beta-carotene and vitamin C, potassium and fiber, apricots also supply phytonutrient carotenoids, including lycopene.

Apricot kernel oil is high in beta-carotene and B vitamins and is considered beneficial for the skin. It makes a good massage oil during pregnancy, when it's best to avoid most essential oils, and features in many stretch-mark products since it soothes inflammation and rejuvenates skin cells. This very emollient oil suits even sensitive and dry skin, and because of its light texture, is easily absorbed.

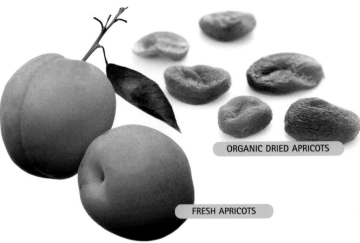

ORGANIC DRIED APRICOTS

FRESH APRICOTS

STRETCH MARK OIL

Essential oils are generally contraindicated during pregnancy until the third trimester, though those recommended here are considered generally safe in the final few weeks. Neroli, or orange flower, oil is good for stress, anxiety, and fear; mandarin is uplifting and soothes the nervous system.

2 tbsp apricot kernel oil
2 tbsp grapeseed oil
1 tsp argan or rosehip oil
1 vitamin E capsule
4 drops each essential oil of neroli and mandarin in the weeks immediately prior to birth

Place the oils in a bowl, prick the capsule, squeeze in and stir well to combine. In the final weeks add either one or both of the essential oils, stirring well before use. Warm a little oil between your palms, then massage around the tops of your thighs and buttocks, and the sides of your waist, stroking in a clockwise direction toward the heart. If you can't reach, instruct your partner!

QUICK AND EASY DISHES

- *Rehydrate dried apricots overnight, then serve with creamy Greek yogurt and a handful of seeds for breakfast.*
- *Whiz up apricots with banana and yogurt for a morning smoothie.*
- *Ready-to-eat apricots can be added to homemade muesli for a filling start to the day.*

BUYING NOTES

Buy fresh apricots only if they are plump and deep orange in color—sniff them too; if they lack scent they probably won't taste good. It can be hard to find perfectly ripe, tasty apricots in stores, although they may be available from farmers' markets. If you are lucky enough to have a tree, pick when fully ripe: Austrian research suggests antioxidant levels rise as fruit ripens.

Favor dried apricots over hard, lemon-colored fresh ones. Bright orange dried apricots may have been treated with sulfur dioxide and sulfites, which can cause a reaction if you are asthmatic. It's best to buy darker brown unsulfured or organic dried apricots.

CULINARY DOS AND DON'TS

- Eat with iron-rich foods to make the iron more accessible.
- Cut fresh apricots into pancakes.
- Add dried apricots to Middle Eastern stews, with lamb or chicken.

apricots

POMEGRANATES

In Arabic lore, the pomegranate is associated with the nurturing qualities of the mother's breast, and in Greek mythology with the mothering goddess Demeter, while the Old Testament command to "be fruitful and multiply" is linked in Jewish thought with the pomegranate. This jewel-colored fruit is considered one of the most antioxidant there is, and in Iran, the world's most prolific producer, pomegranates are highly recommended during pregnancy.

GOOD FOR YOU AND YOUR BABY
A rich source of beta-carotene, vitamins E and C (a single fruit provides about 40 percent of daily requirements), vitamin B_6, and folate, pomegranates also contain potassium and fiber. There are three times more antioxidant phenolic compounds (including tannins, anthocyanins, and ellagic acid) in pomegranate juice than in green tea or red wine, both of which are not recommended in pregnancy. The compounds may minimize cell damage and improve immune function and blood flow, keep arteries from thickening, lower blood pressure, and

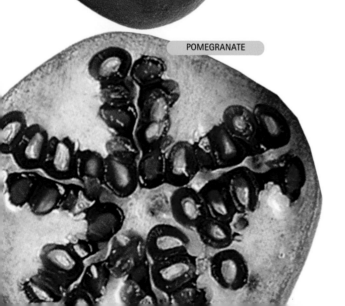

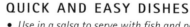

block inflammation. A study in *Pediatric Research* linked drinking pomegranate juice in pregnancy with increased protection of newborns' brains following oxygen deficiency during birth. A University of Colorado study has suggested it may also lessen the effect of high altitude exposure on pregnant women and their babies. In Spain the juice is recommended to ease upset stomachs and wind. It also has antiviral and antibacterial properties. Body lotions containing oil extracted from the seeds by cold-pressing are useful for restoring elasticity to very dry skin.

Like grapefruit juice, pomegranate juice seems to interact with some medication, particularly those for lowering blood pressure; check with your doctor and don't drink more than 1½ cups daily. Avoid pomegranate skin during pregnancy.

BUYING NOTES
Look for dark red or pink skin. The heaviest fruit contain the most seeds. Don't worry about ugly-looking skin, but avoid any with cracks or bruising.

Fruit are ripest in midwinter.

CULINARY DOS AND DON'TS
- To reach the pulpy seeds, break through the leathery skin and bitter membrane. Either slice the fruit almost in half and open with your fingers over a bowl of water (the seeds will sink) or cut into six sections and scoop out the seeds with your fingers. Be aware that the juice stains.
- To juice the seeds, pulse in a blender until liquefied, then strain through cheese cloth; sweeten to taste.
- To catch the juice, roll the fruit until the seeds burst inside, then stick in a straw and hold over a bowl.

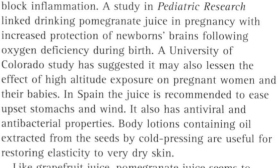

QUICK AND EASY DISHES
- *Use in a salsa to serve with fish and poultry.*
- *Add the seeds as a garnish to sweet and savory salads, main courses, and desserts .*
- *Bake the seeds in muffins.*
- *Serve as an accompaniment to cheeses.*
- *Use as a souring agent in Middle Eastern dishes.*

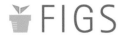 # FIGS

Though dried figs are available year-round, the fresh fruit is a real treat—at once perfumed, chewy, and crunchy. Figs have been associated since ancient times with fertility and nursing—Roman mythology links them with the mother wolf who raised Romulus and Remus. Keep some in your bag and/or locker to stave off cravings and nausea.

Fig trees are relatively easy to grow except in the coldest of climates, and do well in pots.

GOOD FOR YOU AND YOUR BABY

Figs are a fine source of minerals, including potassium and manganese, plus a little calcium, magnesium, iron, and zinc—a mix said to resemble human breastmilk.

Dried figs supply vitamin B_6 and omega-3 fatty acids, and are high in fiber. The dried fruit especially acts as a gentle laxative.

BUYING NOTES

Fresh figs should be plump, well-colored and soft (but not mushy) and have a perfumed scent. Buy ready to eat rather than to store: Austrian research shows that the ripest fruit contains most antioxidants. Farmers' markets are more likely to supply types with variegated-colored skin and flesh, from purple-black to amber. Choose organic dried figs to avoid exposing yourself to sulfur compounds, especially if you have asthma.

CULINARY DOS AND DON'TS

- Chop into morning muesli or anytime yogurt.
- Eat the ripe fresh fruit skin and all.
- Simmer dried figs in a little fruit juice for a few minutes to make them plumper.

QUICK AND EASY DISHES

- *Whiz up with banana and yogurt for a filling shake.*
- *Mix quartered figs, crumbled feta, toasted walnuts with chopped mint. Dress with fruity olive oil for a tasty salad.*
- *Brush honey over the cut sides of fig halves and broil. Serve with toasted almonds and Greek yogurt for a delicious dessert.*

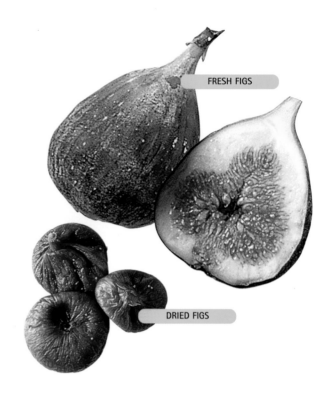

FRESH FIGS

DRIED FIGS

In the Indian tradition, women who eat figs during pregnancy are thought to have shorter labors and recover more speedily after birth.

FIG FLOWER

An attractive way to serve figs is to open them up so you can see the inside. If you desire, you can spoon or pipe a filling into the center. Trim the stalk end with a knife. Cut a deep cross in the top of the fig and open it out by pushing the sides slightly with your fingers.

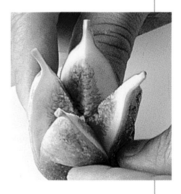

figs

WALNUTS

In Chinese lore, eating walnuts during pregnancy guarantees a brainy child. There may be some truth in this, since the nuts are very rich in the omega-3 fatty acids so essential for brain development. Walnuts have long been connected with fertility: in ancient Rome they were thrown at weddings to augur a quick pregnancy, and in France, a bountiful walnut tree in the garden is said to indicate an abundance of mother's milk in the home. Just four walnuts a day provide a healthy amount of omega-3 fatty acids; make this a priority if you don't eat fish.

GOOD FOR YOU AND YOUR BABY

One of the best sources of antioxidants, including vitamin E, selenium, and the phenolic compound ellagic acid, walnuts also contain manganese and copper and are an excellent source of omega-3 fatty acids. Studies suggest that walnuts may be even more useful in improving heart health than olive oil; the constituent amino acid L-arginine promotes elasticity of the blood vessels, helping to lower high blood pressure. They will be useful once you have a baby: in a University of Texas study, eating walnuts correlated with increased melatonin in the blood, and melatonin promotes sleep.

Don't worry about putting on weight; in a large Spanish study, people who ate nuts at least twice a week were less likely to put on weight than those who did not. A good proportion of the fat is monounsaturated.

Walnut oil adds emollience in massage oil blends for dry skin and is considered useful for stretch marks (do a patch test if you suffer nut allergies). It is reputed to heal skin conditions such as eczema and fungal

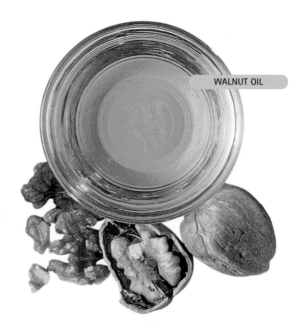

WALNUT OIL

Walnuts are both nutritious and versatile. Along with pecans they can act as a substitute for most nuts in numerous recipes, from desserts to dinners and salads.

infections while promoting skin regeneration and the healing of wounds.

BUYING NOTES

Choose the heaviest dried nuts and avoid ready cracked nuts, which go rancid quickly. "Wet" walnuts are available earlier in the season. Not yet dried, they have a creamy taste and texture. The best walnuts are preserved by sun-drying; these last longer than those preserved by other means. Hunt out white and black walnuts in farmers' markets; the black ones are more pungent and the white ones sweeter and oilier on the palate than ordinary walnuts.

CULINARY DOS AND DON'TS

- Substitute walnut oil for regular oils in stir-fries and salads.
- Chop and sprinkle on pancakes, with maple syrup.
- Add to creamy cheeses (in studies, walnuts seem to mop up fat).
- The astringent flavor works well with young spinach leaves and ripe pear.
- Bake in cakes and loaves.
- Look for walnut butter blends.
- Make a pesto of wet walnuts in a mortar and pestle to serve over chicken or pasta.

QUICK AND EASY DISHES

- *For a delicious light meal, cook tagliatelle with steamed broccoli and chopped walnuts. Add a lemon-olive oil dressing and ground pepper .*
- *Put some chopped walnuts, along with lightly cooked onions, green and red peppers in a frittata to give it added texture.*
- *Create a tasty hummus using peppers and toasted walnuts. Have with pitta bread or raw vegetables for a quick lunch.*

ALMONDS

The most nutritionally dense of all nuts, almonds are another plant long associated with a healthy pregnancy, given as a token of fertility and abundance at weddings in the Middle East and Europe and in the Indian tradition said to bring about an intelligent child.

GOOD FOR YOU AND YOUR BABY

A handful of almonds provides a super dose of manganese, vitamin E, magnesium, vitamin B_2, and phosphorus, plus a little copper, potassium, and calcium. Almonds are a great source of protein—more than an egg!—and fiber, plus monounsaturated fats. The manganese and copper work in tandem to raise energy levels while the vitamin E and potassium together protect against high blood pressure. In one study, the more almonds consumed in a meal, the less high the subsequent rise in blood-sugar. Eat the skin: according to a study in the *Journal of Nutrition*, it contains a unique combination of flavonoids which reacts with the vitamin E to more than double the antioxidant load. Almonds may have a prebiotic effect, supporting the health of the gastrointestinal tract.

Sweet almond oil is one of the most popular base oils for massage. It is quite oily, which feels good on dry, itchy skin, and is recommended in Ayurvedic and

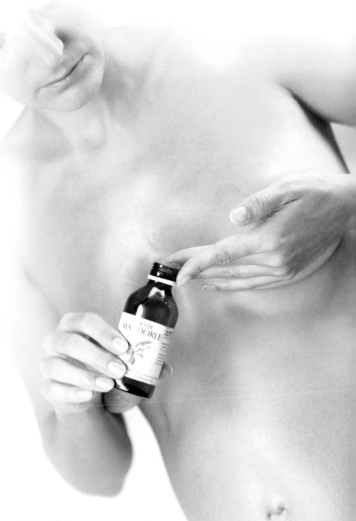

traditional Chinese medicine for eczema and psoriasis. Use to massage the perineum in the six weeks or so before birth for 5–15 minutes to guard against tearing. Avoid if you have a nut allergy.

BUYING NOTES

For keeping, buy almonds in the shell, making sure the shell is whole and not discolored. Smell shelled almonds before use to check for rancidity.

CULINARY DOS AND DON'TS

- Roast and serve with a little sea salt to avoid the additives in processed almond snacks.
- Add to stir-fries.
- Can be eaten as almond butter.
- Look for cake recipes based on ground almonds.
- Use the oil in salad dressings.

NATURAL MAKEUP REMOVER

Suiting all skin types, this is a gentle, all-natural cleanser. However, if you are allergic to nuts, do not use. This recipe makes enough for about one week. Drop the oil on a soft cotton pad and gently wipe over your face to remove makeup. To remove excess oil before applying your cleanser, soak a clean face cloth in warm water, squeeze well and wipe across the skin.

6 tbsp sweet almond oil
6 drops essential oil of neroli

Pour the almond oil into a sterilized dark glass bottle. Drop in the essential oil of neroli. Replace the lid and store in a cool dark place. Shake before use.

AVOCADOS

In Aztec communities, virgins were once warned not to venture outside during the avocado harvest for fear of being made pregnant by the paired fruit of this "testicle" tree! Today, the comforting texture and buttery flavor of avocados seems to tempt the palate when other foods bring on queasy sensations. Get used to buying them now, since they make a perfect first baby food.

GOOD FOR YOU AND YOUR BABY

A good source of vitamin K and potassium (more than a banana), folate, vitamins B_6 and C, and copper, the flesh is some 25 percent protein and is also a source of fiber and monounsatuated fats. The antioxidant carotenoid alpha-carotene seems to reduce cholesterol.

Deep green viscous avocado oil suits facial massage—it is fine-textured and nourishing, helping to maintain tone. Try it over flaky, dry areas. If you suffer skin breakouts during pregnancy, applying mashed avocado can soothe and cool; it is valued by herbalists for its ability to "draw." Avocado has long been used as a hair pomade, to add shine and stimulate growth. (Avoid the oil if you are latex-sensitive.)

Do not eat the anise-flavored leaves, a delicacy in some parts of Latin America; they have an abortifacient action (abortifacients can cause miscarriage).

BUYING NOTES

Choose avocados that are already soft enough to eat. Look for darker skins and press them; they should give way but not cave in. Harder fruit can be ripened at home, but may rot before it is edible. Store in a brown paper bag or next to bananas to speed ripening. Hass are best known but Fuerte are also available, as are Reed, a fully round summer variety with a creamy taste.

QUICK AND EASY DISHES

- *Halve and remove the pit, then pour 1 tsp of balsamic vinegar into the cavity, with salt and black pepper; eat with a teaspoon.*
- *Mix together chopped avocado, cherry tomatoes, and cilantro, add half of a finely chopped red chile and lime juice. Serve as a side with grilled salmon.*

CULINARY DOS AND DON'TS

- To pit an avocado, cut it lengthwise in half all aroud the pit. Twist the halves in opposite directions until separated. Carefully strike the pit with a chef's knife. Twist to dislodge the pit.
- Add to salads and sandwiches at the last minute or the flesh will turn gray.
- Avocado is usually better raw than cooked.
- The flavors work best with shrimp and lime juice, or with basil, mozzarella, and ripe tomatoes.
- After slicing into salads, sprinkle with lemon or lime juice to stop the flesh oxidizing.

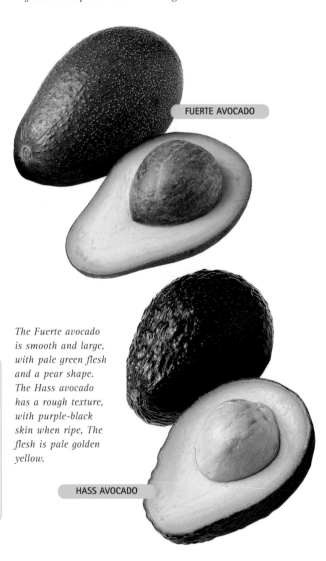

FUERTE AVOCADO

The Fuerte avocado is smooth and large, with pale green flesh and a pear shape. The Hass avocado has a rough texture, with purple-black skin when ripe, The flesh is pale golden yellow.

HASS AVOCADO

OLIVES

Now most often associated with a Mediterranean diet, olive trees were once a symbol of fecundity, able to flourish and bear fruit in the most barren conditions. They were sacred to the Greek goddess Athene. Though olive oil has been found responsible for lowered blood pressure, much of the trumpeted health benefits of the Mediterranean way of eating derive from its focus on many fruits and vegetables, legumes, and whole grains.

GOOD FOR YOU AND YOUR BABY

Olives contain iron and copper, but are best known for their monounsaturated fatty acids (which are 75 percent oleic acid) and extremely high dose of antioxidants, including vitamin E, chlorophyll, and the phytonutrient carotenoids and phenolic compounds, which have anti-inflammatory, antioxidant, and anticoagulant properties. They support the blood vessels' ability to relax and dilate, guarding against high blood pressure, and also reduce blood-clotting. The phenolic compounds also seem to be good for bone health, have an antimicrobial action on food-borne pathogens, and appear to settle gastrointestinal problems.

The stinging sensation at the back of the throat in peppery extra-virgin olive oil indicates the presence of oleocanthal; it has pain-relieving and anti-inflammatory powers similar to ibuprofen.

Olive oil makes a lovely massage oil, traditionally
used to counter stretch marks as well
as for ritual anointing.

Once you get over the stickiness and pungency, olive oil can be helpful for acne and dry skin. Its constituent unsaturated fatty acid squaline occurs naturally in human skin, and is thought useful for boosting suppleness and countering environmental damage.

BUYING NOTES

Choose extra-virgin olive oil for maximum antioxidants (and finest flavor), favoring opaque containers such as cans and dark bottles to preserve maximum phenolic compounds. Use oil within 12 months, since phytonutrients are lost in keeping.

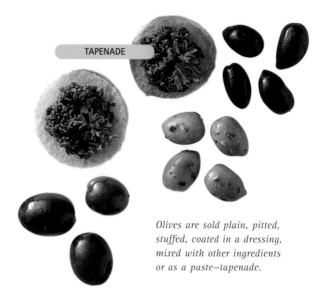

TAPENADE

Olives are sold plain, pitted, stuffed, coated in a dressing, mixed with other ingredients or as a paste—tapenade.

Olives are considered of best nutritional value when bought fresh and loose or packed in oil, rather than cured in brine. Those with pits are finer in flavor than pitted, filled, or marinated varieties.

Green and black olives are not different varieties; the green ones are unripe and the black have been ripened on the tree—you hope (some cheaper pitted olives have been chemically colored or oxidized). Look for named varieties for best taste: Italian Gaeta, French Picholine, and Spanish Manzanilla.

CULINARY DOS AND DON'TS

- Serve a saucer of fine olive oil at table for dipping, rather than butter for spreading.
- Make dressings with olive oil and balsamic vinegar.
- Add olive oil to dishes throughout the day to build up positive health properties.
- Eat at lunchtime to keep blood-sugar levels stable in the afternoon.
- Substitute olive oil for butter in potato dishes.
- Use to stir-fry broccoli: in studies this preserved vitamin C and phenolic compounds over other oils.

QUICK AND EASY DISHES

- *To make tapenade, pit black (or green) olives, then whiz in a blender with garlic, lemon juice, and olive oil; serve on toast.*
- *Add a splash of olive oil, along with some salt and pepper, to boiled potatoes that have been slightly mashed.*

olives

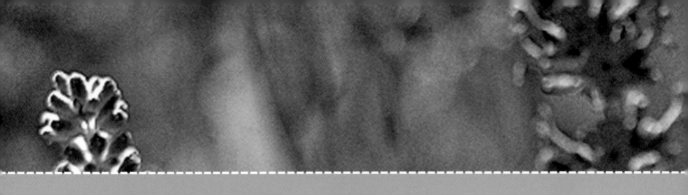

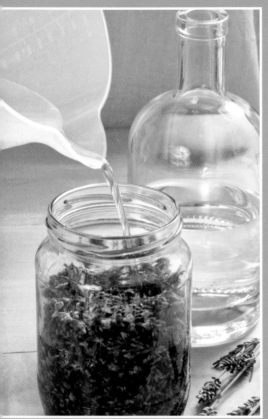

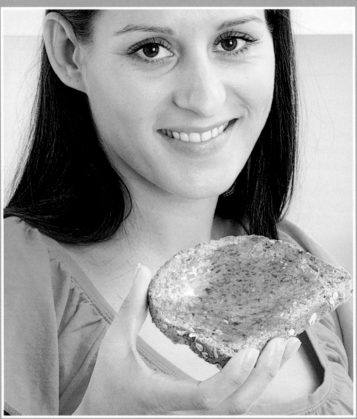

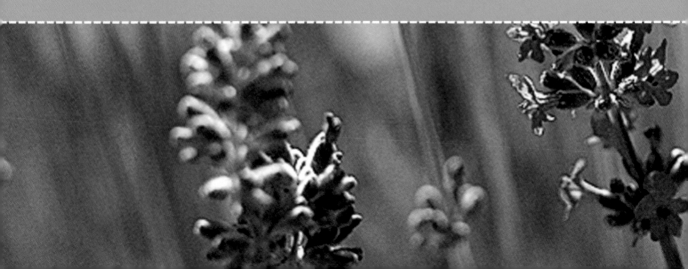

SUSTENANCE FROM THE FLOWER BED

Learn the art of relaxation: it is not a luxury but a daily necessity during pregnancy, helping to safeguard both your well-being and your baby's health. Studies show that stress seems more troubling in the first trimester and after the birth, so do try to relax more during these weeks. What could be more perfect than relaxing with a book in a plant-filled garden or patio or being lulled to sleep by its scents and sounds surrounded by plants that look good and do you good?

JERUSALEM ARTICHOKES • SUNFLOWERS
HONEY • LAVENDER

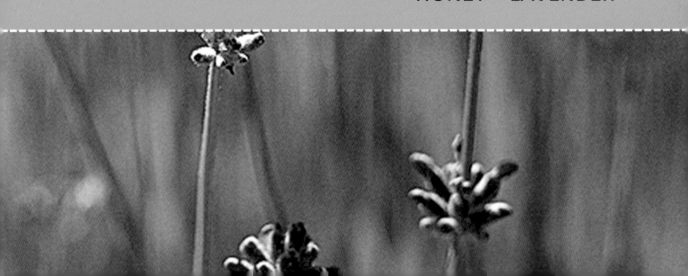

JERUSALEM ARTICHOKES

A Native American crop with bright yellow flowers, "sun roots" can be planted at the back or center of a border to create a tall summer screen. They look like sunflowers, hence another moniker "sunflower artichoke," but thankfully during pregnancy are much easier to grow. The tasty tubers are ready to eat from the fall and have a delicate, smoky taste and good amounts of pregnancy-essential minerals.

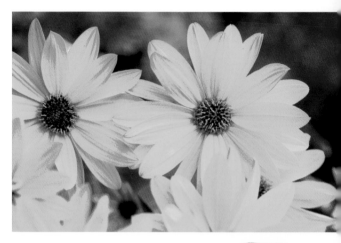

GOOD FOR YOU AND YOUR BABY

A great source of potassium (six times the amount of a banana), plus iron, magnesium, copper and phosphorus, vitamins B and C, and folate, Jerusalem artichokes contain protein and fiber, too. The nutrient load lies just beneath the skin. Much of the tuber is formed by the starch inulin, which not all of us can tolerate and which is to blame for the tuber's much famed ability to cause wind. If pregnancy is making you windy already, start by eating small amounts. Jerusalem artichokes contain prebiotic fructooligosaccharides (FOS)—food for friendly bacteria in the digestive tract—and support the growth of natural probiotics, helpful bacteria, in the digestive tract. This can help reduce bowel upsets.

BUYING NOTES

Jerusalem artichokes are not widely available in supermarkets as they are difficult to harvest mechanically and don't travel or store well. You are more likely to find them at farmers' markets and allotment sales. Avoid those that have sprouted or are tinged green.

GROWING AND HARVESTING NOTES

A member of the sunflower family, the plant thrives in almost any soil and with little tending. Throw a handful of tubers (or parts of) into the ground in spring, stake in

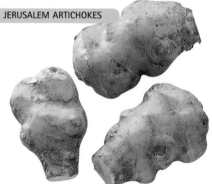

JERUSALEM ARTICHOKES

Jerusalem artichokes have light brown skins, though they can be tinged red or yellow, depending on the conditions. A well-scrubbed artichoke can be eaten raw if thinly grated.

early summer and wait for the 6 foot screen to flourish in late summer and fall. Use tubers from a farmers' market or a neighbor's plot (they aren't generally available in garden centers).

Dig up from after the flowers appear. The tubers keep in the ground well into early spring, and taste better after a frost, when the starch is more digestible. Mark the spot in the fall so you know where to find them.

CULINARY DOS AND DON'TS

- Scrub well under running water to remove soil, especially around the knobbles. Try not to peel: the nutrients lie under the skin.
- Cut into slices before boiling, and use plenty of water for maximum inulin removal.
- Serve alongside boiled ham.
- Add to the roasting pan with winter vegetables.
- Substitute for water chestnuts, both raw and sliced, in stir-fries.

QUICK AND EASY DISHES

- *Julienne with carrots and coat with a walnut-oil vinaigrette.*
- *Make a soup if you're not affected by the inulin, with onion, celery, and vegetable stock.*
- *Boil then mash and mix with potatoes and/or parsnips.*

❦ SUNFLOWERS

These cheery-faced flowers are celebrated for banishing gloomy feelings and instilling a sense of optimism and new potential. They are cheering even when the flowers have faded, since the seeds are a source of tryptophan, which boosts serotonin production, improving mood.

GOOD FOR YOU AND YOUR BABY

Highly concentrated nutrition in a shell, sunflower seeds contain significant amounts of vitamin B and E, folate, iron, niacin, manganese, magnesium, copper, selenium, tryptophan, and phosphorus. The also consist of 25 percent protein. The seeds are rich in phytosterols, plant compounds that seem to enhance immunity. Native Americans consider sunflower seeds a gentle yet effective cure for constipation.

Sunflower oil contains linoleic acid, an omega-6 fatty acid, however most of us in the West consume too much—thanks to processed foods—which can increase blood clotting and inflammation and suppress immunity. To improve your ratio of omega-3 fatty acids to omega-6s, reduce your intake of sunflower oil and up your dose of oily fish. Sunflower oil does suit massage, however, being light and non-greasy on the skin.

BUYING NOTES

As the seeds are high in fats, they easily become rancid—choose the freshest you can and smell before use. Store in a sealed jar in a cool, dark place. If buying unshelled, look for firm, unbroken gray-black shells. Cold-pressed sunflower oil is finest.

GROWING AND HARVESTING NOTES

Sunflowers are great for a new garden, since the roots break up compacted soil. But they do best in fertile, manured, well-draining soil, with a long day of

In Native American traditions, the sunflower symbolizes strength and endurance, thus making them a good prelabor snack.

ENERGY-BOOST SEED MIX

Native Americans carried high-energy snack balls on trails. This portable treat is tastier than many sugar-loaded commercial trail mixes and maintains energy when you are far from home and healthy snacks.

2 tbsp each: chopped almonds, chopped hazelnuts, chopped walnuts, sunflower seeds, raisins, chopped dried organic apricots, and chopped dried dates
¼ cup nut butter
¼ cup thick honey
¼ cup sesame seeds

Mix the chopped nuts in a bowl with the sunflower seeds, raisins, and chopped dried fruit. Moisten by stirring in the nut butter and honey, then form into small balls. Roll in sesame seeds to coat and allow to dry on wax paper overnight before storing in an airtight container in a cool, dark place.

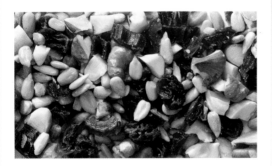

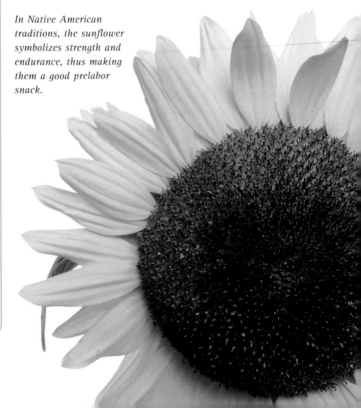

sunshine. The plants are resistant to drought, but water them weekly and mulch well. Companion-plant with squashes for a show and to attract pest-busting predators. Guard young plants against slugs and snails.

Allow the flower heads to dry on the plant—they are ready when the back of the head turns brown and starts to shrivel.

For home-growing, select on habit and appearance, which range from dwarfing to giant, single or double, sunshine yellow to flaming orange or bronze. Native to America, it is always worth tracking down heritage varieties. It is said that women and girls would sing to the young plants like babies, to help them grow.

CULINARY DOS AND DON'TS

- Sunflower seeds taste best when dry-roasted or toasted; this enhances their nutty flavor. Spread the seeds in a thin layer in a small roasting pan, place in

a 325°F oven, and cook for about 4–5 minutes, shaking the pan occasionally.
- Toss the roasted seeds into salads or roasted vegetables just before serving, or mix with a dash of soy sauce.
- Blend a handful in a smoothie.
- Throw ½ cup of seeds into dough when baking bread.

HONEY

It takes a million flowers and 80,000 bees to produce just 1 cup of honey, so the more flowering plants you cultivate to attract the honey-bee, the better, since honey-bees globally are facing colony collapse. They are considered an ancient harbinger of pregnancy. From ancient India and Babylon and in Jewish tradition, honey is as enveloped in pregnancy lore as milk and eggs are, as it is thought to bring luck, fertility, and boy babies to those who eat or drink it. Start the day with a warm lemon juice and honey drink.

To attract bees, cultivate plants that bloom year-round—the easiest way to do this is to be laissez-faire about "weeds" such as dandelions, buttercups, and clover. Bees are traditionally kept to pollinate fruit trees and are attracted to the flowers of strawberries, raspberries, blackberries, currants, and single early flowering roses such as *Rosa rugosa*. They also like blue, yellow and purple flowers, the daisy family, honeysuckle, broom shrubs, and low-growing herbs such as rosemary, lavender, and borage. Avoid flowers bred as doubles (many marigolds and dahlias), which have much less pollen.

GOOD FOR YOU AND YOUR BABY

Honey is comprised of 80 percent natural sugars, which unlike other forms of sugar have been shown to keep blood-sugar levels fairly constant. It also contains traces

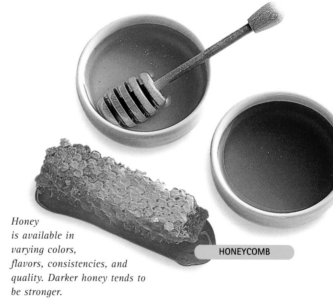

HONEYCOMB

Honey is available in varying colors, flavors, consistencies, and quality. Darker honey tends to be stronger.

of B vitamins, plus calcium, copper, iron, magnesium, manganese, phosphorus, potassium, and zinc. The antioxidant properties derive from pinocembrin, a chemical found only in honey.

Honey is used in hospitals around the world to heal wounds. In trials, cesarean incisions treated with honey healed more cleanly and resulted in less infection and a reduced hospital stay when compared with conventional treatment, while studies in Israeli hospitals suggest it increases patient immunity. Use it on cuts and scrapes to combat bacteria and to keep wounds clean, or use it on your facial skin in case of outbreaks of blemishes.

sustenance from the flower bed

Honey supports friendly bacteria in the digestive tract, too, as different varieties contain varying amounts of lactobacilli and bifidobacteria. Mix a spoonful into warm milk before bed to counter heartburn.
The antimicrobial effect of honey suits the treatment of sore throats and colds; use to sweeten a whole lemon juiced with hot water. A study at Penn State College of Medicine found a spoonful of buckwheat honey as effective in treating children's night-time coughs as conventional cough medicine.

An endurance food, honey is used to improve athletic performance and to counter fatigue; it can help maintain optimal blood-sugar levels through and after training and promote muscle recovery; keep it to hand during labor to sweeten raspberry leaf tea or hot water for instant energy.

Honey is hygroscopic; it absorbs moisture from the air so makes an effective moisturizing face mask.

BUYING NOTES

Phytonutrients are most potent in raw or unpasteurized honey. It's tricky to source "raw" honey at supermarkets, but it's widely available at allotment sales and produce shows. Choose local honey if you get hay fever; many sufferers believe it minimizes the effects of local pollen.

Manuka honey from tea tree flowers in New Zealand is the best-known antimicrobial honey. This doesn't mean your local honey isn't effective; it just hasn't been subject to expensive research studies. Darker honeys, such as buckwheat, sage, tupelo or red gum, and honeydew honeys (made from aphids rather than nectar) are considered more antioxidant and antibacterial. Eucalypt honey is favored by many for relieving colds and sore throats.

CULINARY DOS AND DON'TS

- Many doctors recommend avoiding all unpasteurized products during pregnancy, so check with your doctor before using "raw" honey.
- If honey is too "stiff" to spread, stand the jar in a bowl of hot water.
- When energy flags, spread honey on whole-wheat toast or stir into yogurt.
- Substitute honey for sugar in hot drinks, oatmeal and baking. Because honey is sweeter than sugar use $\frac{1}{2}$–$\frac{3}{4}$ the amount (this may affect cake recipes).
- Never give honey to a baby less than two years old, as it may contain spores of *Clostridium botulinum* and bacteria that can cause botulism.

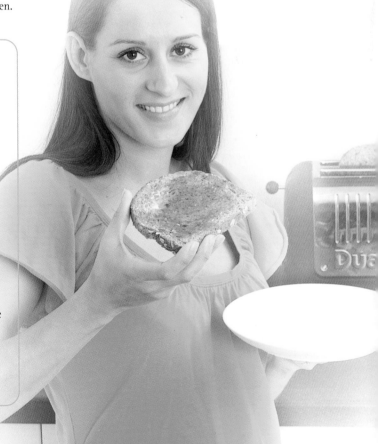

FACE MASK FOR DRY SKIN

This leaves the skin smooth and boosts relaxation, if only because you've rested for 20 minutes. Orange blossom water is associated with romance and fertility.

1 small ripe avocado
1 tbsp honey
2–4 tbsp orange blossom water
1–2 tsp rosehip oil

Scoop the avocado flesh into a bowl and mix in the honey. Secure your hair away from your face and cleanse away makeup. Apply the mask, smearing it over your face and neck, then recline for 10–15 minutes, supported by pillows. Wipe away the debris with an old clean face cloth, then splash your face with lukewarm water. Dampen a clean cloth with the orange blossom water and wipe away any last traces of the mask. Moisturize your whole face with the rosehip oil, if desired.

MAKING LAVENDER WATER

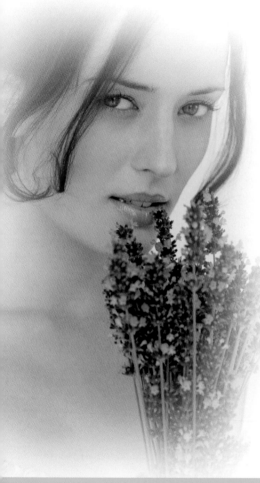

During your third trimester add a little of this uplifting but calming scented water to the final rinse in your washing machine for its clean aroma, use in the iron when pressing bed linen to encourage sleep, or use to spritz kitchen worktops to kill germs. If you are not using your own lavender grown without pesticides, choose dried organic lavender. Do not use the tincture directly on your skin.

You will need:

Large lidded glass jar
3½ oz lavender flowers (weight of flowers when removed from stem)
1 cup vodka
1 cup distilled water
Clean dark glass bottle with a lid

1 Place the lavender flowers into the large glass jar. Pour over the vodka and then the distilled water, making sure that the flowers are covered by at least 2 inches of liquid. You may need to add more vodka and water to achieve this. Lid and leave in a cool, dark place for one month. Shake every few days.

2 After 1 month, strain the liquid through cheese cloth into a bowl and, wearing surgical gloves, squeeze the cloth to extract as much liquid as possible. Discard the cheese cloth and lavender flowers.

3 Using a funnel, decant the lavender water into the clean, dark glass bottle and lid tightly. Store in a cool, dark place.

4 To use the water, pour into the reservoir of your iron, add a little to the washing machine before the final rinse, or decant into a spritzer bottle and top up with water. Shake before spraying.

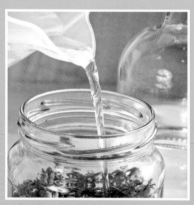

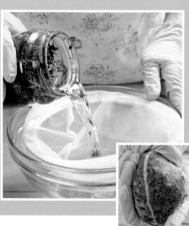

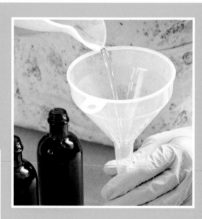

☘ LAVENDER

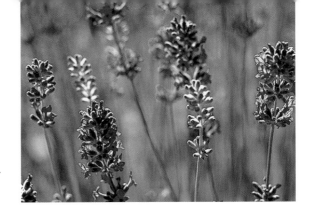

Grown outside windows and doors or to edge beds, lavender transfers its scent readily when brushed with the fingertips, and many swear by the relaxing but uplifting aroma for easing physical and mental tension. Although lavender is traditionally recommended in pregnancy to alleviate ailments including insomnia, anxiety and mood swings, it is a uterine stimulant, so avoid the essential oil and herbal remedies in the first trimester and high doses throughout pregnancy. The National Association for Holistic Aromatherapy in the United States advises avoiding the oil completely until the postpartum period.

GOOD FOR YOU AND YOUR BABY

Research confirms that lavender has calming, soothing and sedative properties and is antibacterial and antiviral. The oil has been effective in easing stress, anxiety and insomnia, reversing hair loss, and treating postoperative pain. In one study, bathing with lavender oil was more effective in relieving pain in the perineum following birth than a placebo. Lavender is also used in massage oils, inhalations, infusions and tinctures to relieve headaches and muscle tension, treat indigestion, bloating and wind, skin conditions, to lift exhaustion and negative moods, and to boost mental performance.

Talk to your doctor before using lavender if taking antidepressants.

BUYING NOTES

Choose best-quality essential oil in dark glass bottles and use within six months. Check when buying dried flowers that they are labelled with their botanical name.

Lavandula angustifolia (aka English lavender or true lavender) yields the best-quality oil and is expensive. The hybrid *Lavandula x intermedia* (lavandin) produces more but less medicinally desirable oil (it is generally used for laundry products). *Lavandula latifolia* (spike or Spanish lavender) is of lesser quality and duly less expensive. Bottles which are marked "lavender oil" are adulterated or blends.

GROWING AND HARVESTING NOTES

Because this is a Mediterranean shrub, it thrives in sunny, free-draining conditions, is drought resistant, and tolerates poorer soil and a little cold, but not excessive damp. It suits window boxes, large pots, and neglectful pregnancy gardeners. When growing your own, raise the cultivar *Lavandula angustifolia*, "Hidcote".

Plant young plants in late spring—1 foot apart for a hedge or wider for bushes—and prune to encourage plants to bush out. Be warned that cutting below the last piece of live foliage into old wood kills a branch. Prune the heads after flowering.

Much of the volatile oil (which accounts for the refreshing scent and medicinal effects) is found in the flowers. To dry flowers at home, pick in mid to high summer in the morning toward the end of the flowering period, when the lower petals have begun to dry. Hang the stems until dry, then store in an airtight container in a cool, dark place.

DOS AND DON'TS

- Spritz bed linen with lavender water before ironing.
- Make lavender bags and store between clothing to deter moths.
- Fill a pillow with dried flowers to promote sleep and a better mood on waking.
- After the birth, promote sleep and a good mood by adding 5 drops of essential oil combined with 1 tbsp carrier oil in your night-time bath.

HEALING SITZ BATH

Use this to soothe the perineum and encourage healing after the birth.

5 drops essential oil of lavender
5 drops essential oil of sandalwood

Add the oils to a sitz bath or bucket of warm water and swish well. Sit in the water for as long as is comfortable or convenient. Alternatively, add 5 drops essential oil of lavender to a basin of hot water and swish well. Soak a clean cloth in the water, wring out well and apply as a compress.

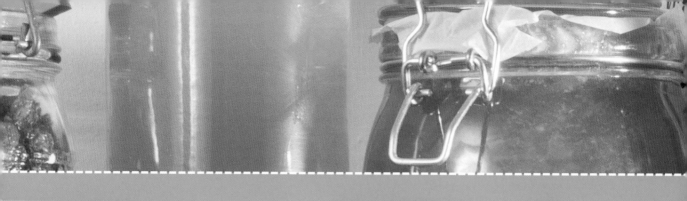

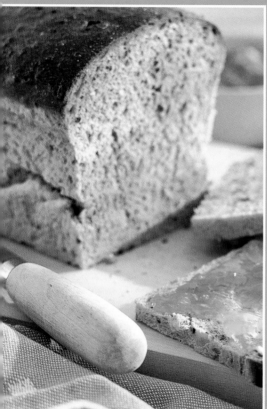

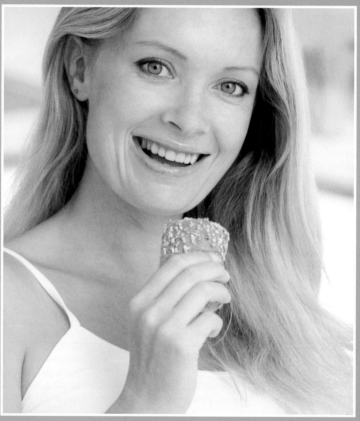

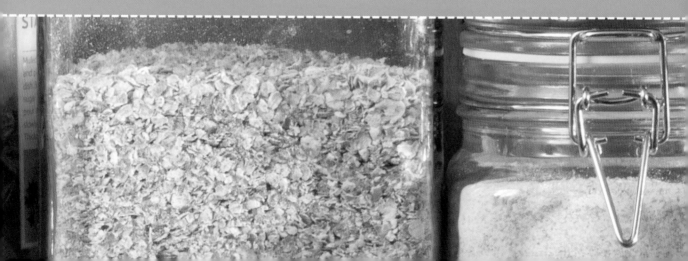

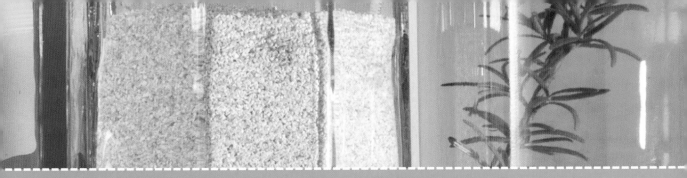

ESSENTIAL PANTRY STAPLES

When the urge to nest strikes, make sure your kitchen cabinets are filled with these whole foods, which will keep for months. Their mix of protein and fiber, iron and B vitamins is important to maintain your energy levels and a calm mood through the long weeks of physical change and emotional uncertainty. If you find it tiring to trek around the supermarket, bulk-buy online, taking advantage of delivery direct to your doorstep.

CHICKPEAS · LENTILS · OATS
RICE · WHOLE WHEAT

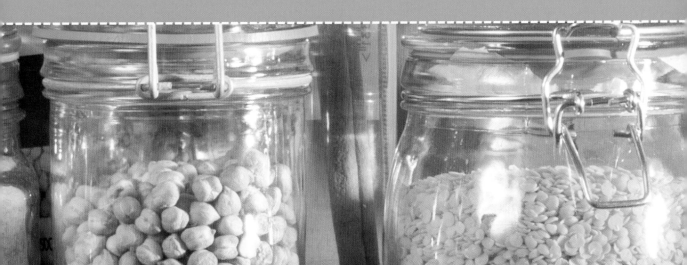

CHICKPEAS

Handy pantry staples, especially for expectant vegetarians, these nutty, buttery legumes can be bought dried in bags or ready to use in cans. They originated in the Middle East, so to find perfect flavor combinations think of other products popular in the region: lemon and garlic, olive oil and sesame paste, mint and yogurt.

GOOD FOR YOU AND YOUR BABY
Chickpeas contain significant amounts of folate and good amounts of copper, iron, and phosphorus. They are excellent sources of manganese and the trace mineral molybdenum, which helps to undo the negative effects of sulfites used as preservatives. Chickpeas are a good source of protein, important for strict vegetarians, and of fiber, which is helpful in easing constipation and keeping blood-sugar levels stable. Chickpeas are rich in phytonutrient saponins and fructooligasaccharides (FOS), both of which seem to be cholesterol-lowering.

BUYING NOTES
Available canned in most supermarkets, ethnic stores and Mediterranean delis are good sources of dried chickpeas sold in packs; check the date if you think the store does not have a fast turnover of stock. Canning reduces the folate by up to 45 percent, so it's best to soak dried beans.

In Mediterranean and Mexican markets you may stumble across this year's early crop: tiny, pale green pods with light green chickpeas inside. They taste tender and delicate—fine eating if you can track them down. Alternatively you may be offered this year's new dried crop, which only require about 90 minutes' cooking.

When buying chickpeas, look for whole beans that are a light brown color, odorless, and uniformly sized.

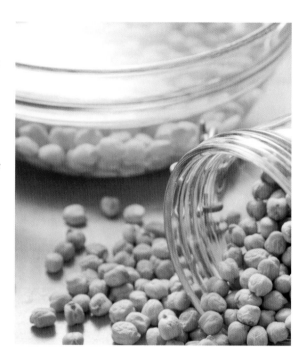

Babies love the creamy texture of chickpeas, and they are chunky enough to pick up in a fist.

QUICK AND EASY DISHES
- *For a quick soup, add 3–4 cans to a sautéed onion and cover with stock. When heated through, blend and add 1 tbsp mint just before serving.*
- *Stir chickpeas into thick yogurt and top with lemon juice and pine nuts; eat with pita.*
- *For a zesty salad, add chopped fresh parsley and mint and plenty of lemon juice and black pepper.*

CULINARY DOS AND DON'TS
- Rinse canned chickpeas thoroughly before use.
- Don't cook canned chickpeas, simply heat through.
- Soak dried beans in plenty of cold water (more than 1 inch higher than the beans) overnight (or for 8 hours) in the refrigerator, then change the water and bring to a boil (don't add salt). Reduce the heat, partially cover the beans and simmer for 1½–3 hours, depending on the recipe, until tender. Skim off scum as it rises to the surface.
- Team chickpeas with dried cumin, turmeric, cilantro.
- Serve with couscous and a piquant sauce.
- If you are vegetarian, serve with brown rice; this provides as good protein as meat or dairy produce.

LENTILS

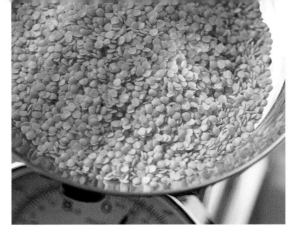

Rich in iron, folate, and protein, lentils are an especially valuable pregnancy food, and are much quicker to prepare than other legumes. You don't have to be a vegetarian to enjoy the perfumed nutty flavor: lentils make wonderfully comforting soups on winter days and creamy dahl curries.

GOOD FOR YOU AND YOUR BABY

An excellent source of manganese and folate containing very useful amounts of iron, phosphorus, copper, B vitamins, and potassium, lentils have the most protein of any legume. They are 25 percent protein and are high in fiber, too, helping counter constipation, benefiting heart health and keeping blood-sugar levels stable. Lentils are an excellent way to take in molybdenum, which helps to undo the effect of sulfites used as preservatives. They also contain isoflavones, organic compounds which help to maintain bone strength.

BUYING NOTES

Some varieties are available in most supermarkets while ethnic and Mediterranean specialty stores may offer a wider variety. Check the date on dried packs if the store does not have a quick turnover. The flavor of canned lentils is disappointing.

Think beyond brown: lentils come in a rainbow of colors—red, yellow, orange, green, even black—and may be lens-shaped or round, large or small, and sold whole or in halves. Fifty varieties are used in Indian cooking,

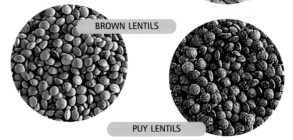

Lentils are extremely nutritious and have been used for thousands of years. They come in many different colors, sizes, and shapes.

GREEN LENTILS

BROWN LENTILS

PUY LENTILS

each with its own name and recommended dishes. Puy lentils have a fine earthy flavor.

QUICK AND EASY DISHES

- *For dahl, simmer red lentils in 3 times their volume of water for 30 minutes. Meanwhile, fry garlic and ginger with mustard and cumin seeds and turmeric; add a chopped onion and fry until soft. When the lentils are soupy (you may need to add more hot water), pour over the spiced fried onion and beat over a low heat or blend until thick.*
- *Refrigerate leftover dahl; next day beat in an egg and freshly chopped onion, then roll into balls and fry; serve with yogurt.*

CULINARY DOS AND DON'TS

- Pick over dried lentils for small stones and other debris, then rinse before cooking.
- No need to presoak; boil straight from the package.
- To cook, add 2–3 times the amount of boiling water, bring back to a boil and simmer for 15–30 minutes.
- Team lentils with onion, garlic, and herbs or spices.
- Use small orange or yellow lentils for dahl curries and soups.
- Larger green or brown lentils hold their shape after cooking; use them in herby salads.
- If you are a vegetarian, eat lentils with brown rice; this provides as good protein as meat or dairy produce.
- Cook with sources of vitamin C, such as tomatoes or green bell peppers, to maximize iron intake.

OATS

This cultivated grass satisfies many cravings for a food that is soothing and filling in pregnancy—and the peculiar lust for "white" foods that many pregnant women share. That liking is handy, because this is one of the most nutritious grains there is. In Scottish lore, counting the grains of oat on a stalk is said to indicate the number of babies you will have.

GOOD FOR YOU AND YOUR BABY

An excellent source of manganese with very good amounts of selenium, plus vitamin B_1, magnesium and phosphorus, zinc, and vitamin E, oats provide a generous supply of protein and fibre (1 cup has almost double the fiber of one slice of whole-wheat bread). Its soluble fiber beta-glucan has been shown to lower cholesterol and enhance the immune system's reaction to bacterial infection. It also stabilizes blood-sugar levels. Eating oats is associated with a healthy heart and, like other whole grains, with reducing the risk of developing type-2 diabetes. Oats contain antioxidant avenanthramides and lignans, which also support heart health. The bran seems to lower cholesterol.

Herbalists use oats to treat depression, exhaustion, and insomnia, and to aid convalescence following

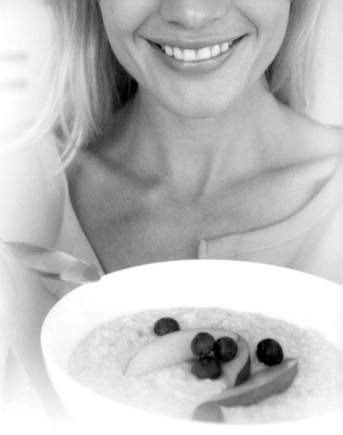

ITCHY SKIN SOAK

To relieve itching and very dry skin, try this bath time herbal remedy. Use the most powdery milled oats you can find (those that dissolve on heating). Add the rose petals once your baby has arrived.

> 1 cup oats
> handful of dried rose petals (optional)
> 1 square cheese cloth

Pile up the oats (and rose petals, if using) in the center of the fabric and tie the ends or secure with an elastic band. Suspend under the hot tap while running a bath. After soaking in the water, rub the bag gently over the affected area, or rub briskly to exfoliate areas of hard skin. Discard after use.

QUICK AND EASY DISHES

- *For a creamy oatmeal add 2½ parts cold milk to 1 part jumbo oats and slowly bring to a boil, stirring often. After the oatmeal has reached the boil, take it off the heat and let sit for 5 minutes. Top with dried fruit, chopped banana or mango, or a sprinkling of cinnamon, or add a few crushed cardamom pods during cooking.*
- *For a delicious dessert, heat a skillet and pour in ¾ cup rolled oats and 1 tbsp sugar. Toast until slightly caramelized and golden. Meanwhile, whip ¾ cup whipping cream, then add to the bowl a drizzle of honey and the juice of 1 lemon and mix together. In a tall glass, layer the oats, ½ cup raspberries, and flavored cream and serve topped with 3 blueberries.*

illness or exertion. A poultice can ease itching skin.
They are also used to help athletes maintain muscle
function and stamina during training sessions. Oats may
help to combat cravings, being used in the treatment of
addiction and as an antismoking aid.

BUYING NOTES

Check the date on dried packs if the store does not have
a quick turnover. Avoid instant oatmeal mixes, which
may contain additives like salt and sugar.

The groat is either cut into pieces ("steel-cut" or
"pinhead" oats) or steamed then rolled flat ("rolled"
oats). Of the rolled oats, jumbo oats are whole steamed
groats and retain their shape and texture during
cooking; quick-cook oats are cut into pieces for speedy
cooking; they aren't nutritionally less useful, just less
satisfying if you like texture. Steel-cut or pinhead oats
have not been steamed, so take longer to cook.

CULINARY DOS AND DON'TS

- The finer the oats, the quicker they cook.
- Substitute for half the flour in a crumble topping.
- Use a bag of oats as a muesli base, adding seeds and
  nuts to taste.
- Sweeten oat dishes with maple syrup or honey.
- Add oat brans to other cereals if you prefer them.
- Snack on oatcakes topped with a sharp hard cheese or
  smoked salmon.

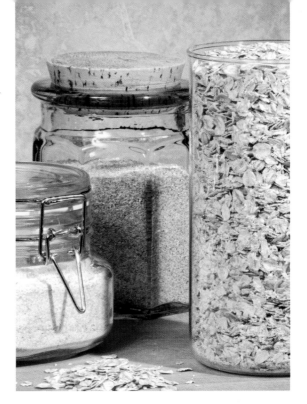

*Oats can be enjoyed in various forms, such as oatbran, rolled
oats, and fine oats. Oatbran and rolled oats can be cooked as
cereals, granola, or ingredients in muffins and bread. Fine
oats are used in instant oatmeal, and if processed into a
powdered form, can be used as baby food.*

RICE

One of the world's most enduring symbols of fertility
and happiness, rice is thrown at weddings across Europe
to augur fertility. In Indonesia, the Rice Mother, Indoea
Padi, is honored and pregnant mothers are offered
glutinous rice cakes, while in India it is ceremonially
given as a baby's first taste of food. In parts of
Malaysia, the wives of rice planters are considered as
worthy of special treatment as a pregnant woman.

GOOD FOR YOU AND YOUR BABY

An excellent source of manganese, and rich in
phosphorus, potassium, and magnesium, rice also
contains essential fatty acids, vitamin E, B vitamins and
iron. The phytonutrient lignans in rice protects against
heart disease and seems to support digestive health, and
its phenolic compounds are antioxidant. Rice is rich in
fiber and becomes a complete protein when served with
lentils or beans. Rice protein seems to improve the
dilation of blood vessels. The high fiber load of brown
rice helps counter constipation, benefits heart health,
and keeps blood-sugar levels stable. It is associated with
a reduced risk of developing type-2 diabetes.

Brown rice (what remains after the hard outer hull of
the grain is removed) is the most nutritious form
because it retains its layer of bran and germ, where the
nutrients cluster. These are removed to make white rice,
and when the grain is then polished to extend shelf life,
the nutritious fatty layer is removed. White rice may be
enriched with the B vitamins and iron it loses in
processing, but still lacks 11 of its original nutrients and
all its fiber.

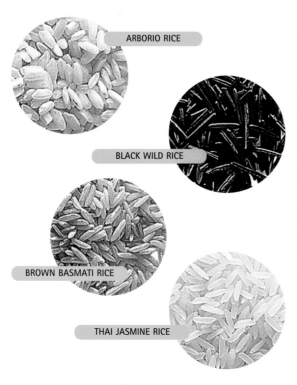

ARBORIO RICE

BLACK WILD RICE

BROWN BASMATI RICE

THAI JASMINE RICE

BUYING NOTES

Brown rice becomes rancid more quickly than polished white rice, so check the sell-by dates if the store does not have a quick turnover. Choose organic or non-US grown rice to avoid pesticide residue: US rice has been found to contain up to five times more arsenic than rice from Europe, India, or Bangladesh. Don't store cooked rice; it is susceptible to fungi growth even when refrigerated, and spoils quickly.

Short-grain rice, such as arborio or sushi, is the most starchy and is best for desserts and sticky dishes, such as risottos and paella. Long-grain rice, such as basmati or Thai jasmine, remains separate in cooking and tends to be served alongside main meals. Search out red, green or black wild rices for their complex flavors. Wild rice is not a true rice but an aquatic grass.

CULINARY DOS AND DON'TS

- Brown rice in hot oil or butter before cooking in stock to help keep grains separate.
- Presoak white and brown long-grain rices, particularly basmati, to speed up cooking time.
- Other than risotto, never stir rice while it cooks; you will break up the holes that allow the steam to escape.
- Team with a lentil or bean dish to activate the protein.

GENTLE RICE CLEANSER

This rice-based cleansing powder is good in the morning and the evening if proprietary cleansers feel harsh or contain chemicals best avoided in pregnancy, such as parabens. If you have a nut allergy, omit the almonds; if you are dairy-intolerant, substitute the milk with orange blossom water.

2 tbsp baby rice
1 tsp ground almonds
2 tbsp whole milk

Mix the rice and almond powders and pour into an airtight jar. Store in a cool, dark place. To use, place a teaspoon or so of powder in the palm of your hand and stir in enough milk to make a smooth paste, adding the liquid little by little and stirring to prevent lumps. Rub into moistened skin, then splash off with warm, then cool water.

QUICK AND EASY DISHES

- To cook brown basmati, add double the amount of cold water to rice (or a little more), stir in a little olive oil and salt, cover and bring to a boil. Once boiled, stir then replace the lid and reduce to the lowest heat and simmer for 45 minutes, covered, checking at intervals to see whether you need more water. Remove from the heat and allow to stand for another 10 minutes.
- Roll your own veggie roll by adding avocado and cucumber slices to a cup of cooked rice on one side of a sheet of nori seaweed, then roll. Sprinkle with sesame seeds.
- Stir chopped vegetables and nuts into cooled rice, then add a tasty dressing.
- Form leftover risotto into balls with a little mozzarella at the center. Fry and serve with a tomato sauce.

WHOLE WHEAT

Another grain associated with mother goddesses, wheat is a dietary staple with a host of health benefits—when unrefined. But in its white, or refined, state it is the cause of many of the developed world's health problems, from obesity and diabetes to cardiovascular disease. It doesn't have to be this way; putting whole-wheat bread and other products at the heart of your daily diet during pregnancy helps to protect you and your baby from future health problems. Start the day with sourdough for long-lasting energy (see page 100).

GOOD FOR YOU AND YOUR BABY

Whole wheat is a fantastic source of folate and B vitamins, vitamin E, zinc, magnesium, and manganese. But when the bran and germ are removed to make white flour, many of the vitamins and minerals and much of the fiber content are lost.

The high fiber load of whole wheat reduces high cholesterol, keeps blood-sugar levels stable, and reduces constipation. Eating whole grains also supports heart health and reduces the risk of developing type-2 diabetes. The phytonutrient lignans in whole wheat protects against heart disease and seems to support gut health, and its phenolic compounds are antioxidant (over 80 percent are found in the germ and bran). People with the highest intake of betaine, a metabolite of choline in wheat, seem to be protected from inflammation.

Many women avoid bread and pasta for fear of weight gain, but in one of the largest studies into women's health (Harvard Medical School/Brigham and Women's Hospital), women who ate whole grains weighed less than those who did not.

BUYING NOTES

Loaves from supermarkets (including their bakeries) and chain bakers are made quickly. This necessitates lots of yeast and sugar, plus all manner of chemical agents and enzymes (which don't have to be listed on the bag) to make the texture palatable and increase shelf life. Leftover yeast in such loaves is not easily digestible, and the additives may not be well tolerated either, leading to bloating and energy dips.

It's best to avoid anything with E-numbers and soy flour, which is tricky in supermarket loaves. Check the label also to see whether healthy-looking brown bread

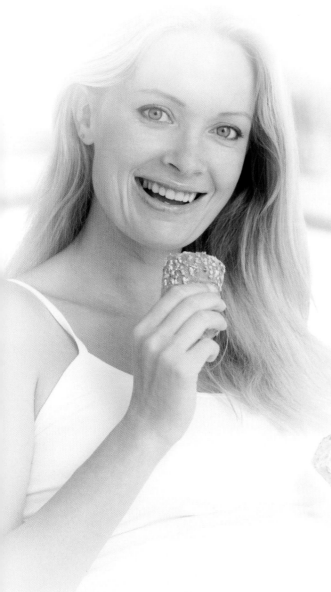

Putting whole-wheat products at the heart of your daily diet helps to protect you and your baby from future health problems.

MAKING A
SOURDOUGH STARTER

Sourdough breads are made without using added yeast; they rise by harvesting yeast in the environment. While the bread-making process is much longer than for regular loaves, to allow for fermentation and the growth of digestion-friendly lactobacilli bacteria, these lend a tangy taste, make available extra nutrients, and preserve the bread naturally. They kill off bad bacteria by creating an acid environment so the loaf stays fresh longer. You need to begin by making a starter, or biga. This seems a long-winded process, but once completed it can live forever. Alternatively, ask your local artisan baker for a little of his or her starter.

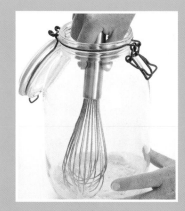

You will need:

bag of organic white bread flour
large bottle of mineral water
tall, wide-mouth glass jar

1 Sterilize the jar by washing in hot soapy water and drying in a low oven. Put ½ cup of the flour and ¼ cup of the water in the jar and stir with a clean metal spoon or whisk. Leave for 24 hours, uncovered, in a warm room (70-80°F).

2 The next day, add the same amount of flour and water again, stir and leave for another 24 hours, covered with plastic wrap with a hole in the top. On the third day, repeat again.

3 On day 4, throw away most of the concoction, leaving a thickish layer in the bottom of the jar. Add double the amount of flour and water to the jar, stir, and leave again.

4 Repeat as for day 4 on day 5, looking for bubbles—a sign of fermentation. Repeat again on day 6, by which time the mixture should have increased in volume.

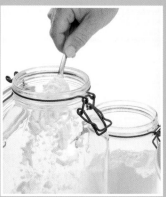

5 Repeat on day 7, or for another week until the starter doubles in size and is frothy on top with bubbles underneath. It should smell sour and yeasty. Your starter is ready to use. If you don't want to use it today, store, covered, in the refrigerator.

6 Use the starter as instructed in a sourdough recipe. The dough will take longer to rise than when using yeast—maybe 2 hours longer. To develop the tangy flavor more, after the first rise, knock back the dough, then cover and let rise in a cool room or refrigerator until doubled in size (up to 2 days in the refrigerator).

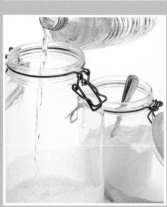

Refreshing the starter
After baking (or weekly), refresh the starter by feeding it with flour and water and throwing it away as before for up to 3 days, until it is nicely frothy again.

is, in fact, made from white flour colored with molasses. Choose organic: because the whole kernel is used, wholegrain products tend to have more pesticide residues than other foods and more than white bread.

The best place to buy bread is from an artisan independent baker, who will have masses of information to share on flours and fermentation methods. Once you find a loaf you love, buy in bulk to freeze. Or, befriend a bread-making machine!

Sourdough bread is a much better source of iron, zinc, and copper than regular bread, and seems to be better tolerated by those with wheat allergies. This may be thanks to the fermentation process, which changes the nature of the starches and adds beneficial bacteria (lactobacillus, as in yogurt) that predigest bran, fight pathogenic organisms, and support healthy intestinal flora. Sourdough's naturally occurring yeast and good bacteria also produce B vitamins and biotin. In one study, those who ate sourdough bread had lower blood-sugar levels than after eating other breads, and the

effects lasted for hours. What performed worst in one study were "whole wheat" breads made from white flour with added germ and bran. Be warned that supermarket sourdough may be made quickly with yeast and added sourdough flavorings.

CULINARY DOS AND DON'TS

- Combine whole wheat with eggs: both are good sources of choline.
- The hassle-free way to home-baked loaves is a bread machine. Set it up before bed to produce a loaf (and scented house) by breakfast time.
- Add dried fruit, nuts, and seeds to your home baking.
- Check flour packaging before buying to avoid bleached flour. Unbleached flour has a light cream color.

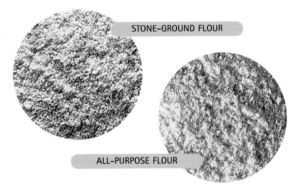

STONE-GROUND FLOUR

ALL-PURPOSE FLOUR

Stone-ground flour retains all of its nutrients through the milling process since all of the wheat kernel is used. Its coarse texture and high nutrition value make it a favorite with bakers. All-purpose flour is a mixture of hard and soft wheats, and contains some protein. It is best used for baking breads, cakes, and pastries.

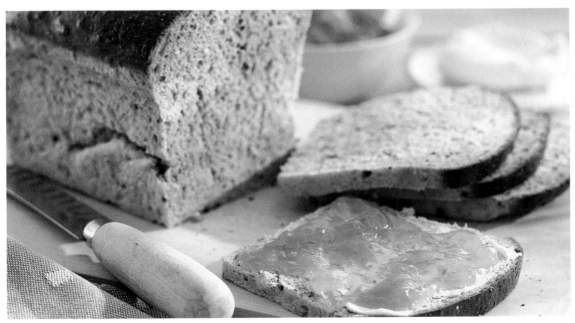

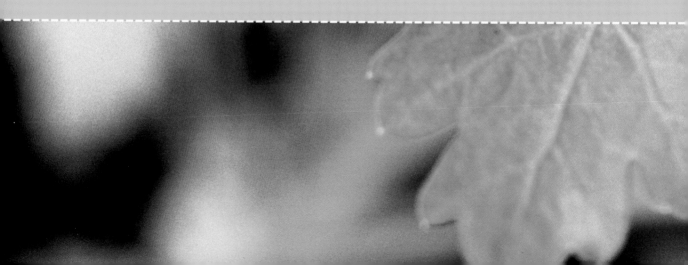
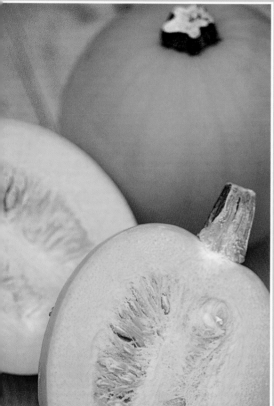
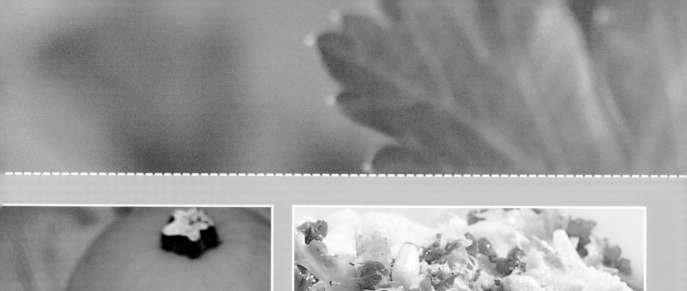
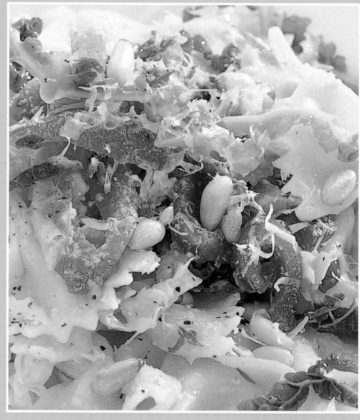

RECIPES

Enjoy the bounty of the seasons, whether from your garden or the supermarket shelves, and create nutrient-rich dishes that will nourish you and your growing baby. As well as tasting delicious, you'll have the satisfaction of knowing that you are creating meals filled with essential vitamins and minerals, which can be enjoyed by all the family. Most are quick and easy to prepare—a boon when you are feeling tired or perhaps a little queasy.

SOUPS · SALADS · EGG DISHES · SHELLFISH · CURRIES · STIR-FRIES
VEGETABLES · SAUCES · BREAD · BREAKFAST CEREALS
PUDDINGS · CRUMBLES · DIPS · PASTA · MEATS
FRUIT DESSERTS · SHAKES

AUTUMN BOUNTY

CREAMY MELON SHAKE

In early fall, when melons are at their ripest, try this yogurt shake containing fruit high in the essential mineral potassium, which helps you to maintain a good fluid balance in pregnancy and counters cramps. It's also packed with calcium and the enzyme superoxide dismutase, which may help to ease symptoms of stress.

preparation time 5 minutes, plus overnight soaking
cooking time 0
serves 2

Contains fiber, protein, potassium, beta-carotene, vitamin C, calcium, phosphorus

2 handfuls of dried apricots, soaked overnight
2 oranges
2 large slices of very ripe cantaloupe or honeydew melon, seeded and cut into chunks
½ cup plain organic yogurt
low-fat organic milk, to taste

• The night before, place the apricots in water to cover and soak overnight.
• The next morning, place the softened apricots, melon chunks, and yogurt in a blender and whiz until well combined.
• Squeeze the oranges and with the motor running, add the juice and enough milk to make a frothy shake runny enough to suit your palate.
• Pour into a glass or over your morning or evening muesli.

FRUITY OATMEAL

Calming oats make a gentle start to the day if you're feeling queasy, and this version is naturally sweetened with apricots for vitamin C and banana for potassium.

preparation time 5 minutes
cooking time 10 minutes
serves 2

Contains fiber, protein, vitamins D, K and C, calcium, manganese, phosphorus, potassium

1 mug jumbo organic oats
2½ mugs lowfat organic milk
8 dried apricots, chopped
8 cardamom pods
1 banana
maple syrup, to serve

• Place the oats, milk, and apricots in a saucepan. In a mortar, crush the cardamom pods with a pestle, then add them to the pan.
• Over a low heat, slowly bring the pan to a boil, stirring constantly. Once the oatmeal is bubbling, take the pan off the heat and leave for 5 minutes to allow the oats to plump up.
• Slice the banana thinly and stir the pieces into the oatmeal.
• To serve, drizzle over maple syrup. For a thinner oatmeal, stir in a little cold milk. Discard the cardamom pods as you find them.

CARROT SOUP

This simple soup is made with chicken stock for a creamy flavor and maximum nutrients, but you can substitute vegetable stock. The soup has few other flavors, so the carrot really shines through. Serve with crusty bread and chunks of sharp cheddar cheese.

preparation time 5 minutes
cooking time 35–40 minutes
serves 2

Contains fiber, protein, beta-carotene, vitamins B and K, manganese

2 tbsp olive oil
1 medium onion, chopped
1 lb organic carrots
1 bay leaf
2½ cups chicken stock (see page 118)
Greek yogurt, to serve

• Pour the olive oil into a large pan, then sweat the thinly sliced onion until soft but not colored.
• Top and tail the carrots, slice them in half lengthwise, then chop into ½ inch slices.
• Add the carrots and bay leaf to the pan and stir until warmed through. Then pour over enough of the stock to cover the carrots.
• Cover and allow to simmer over a medium heat until the carrots are soft, about 20 minutes. Remove the bay leaf. Allow to cool and reserve the pan.
• Place the soup in a blender or food processor and whiz to your desired consistency. If it seems rather thick, add a little boiling water and stir through.
• Pour the soup back into the pan to reheat then serve with a large swirl of Greek yogurt.

MOULES MARINIERES

In early fall, take advantage of the last mussels. They're not only delicious, but packed with vitamins, minerals, protein, and omega-3, and when cooked correctly are perfectly safe in pregnancy. Although the recipe contains wine and cream—the alcohol burns off and it's good to treat yourself occasionally in pregnancy. Serve with fresh crusty bread.

preparation time 10 minutes
cooking time 10 minutes
serves 2

Contains protein, vitamin B_{12}, iron, manganese, selenium, omega-3 fatty acids

  2¼ lb fresh raw mussels
  1 tbsp olive oil
  2–3 shallots, finely chopped
  ⅓ cup white wine
  2 tbsp heavy cream
  1 tbsp chopped fresh parsley

• Discard any broken mussels plus any open mussels that don't close when you tap them sharply. Clean the remaining mussels by pulling away the beard and scraping away barnacles with a sharp knife. Give the mussels a good rinse in a full pan of water, changing the water three times.
• Heat the olive oil in a large pan with a lid that fits tight, then sauté the shallots until soft but not browned, about 2–3 minutes.
• Add the white wine and allow to bubble for 1 minute, uncovered, to burn off the alcohol.
• Add the drained mussels to the pan and put the lid on. Allow to simmer for 3–4 minutes, shaking the pan every now and then, until the mussels open (discard any that don't).
• Stir in the cream and parsley, then ladle the mussels with some of the fragrant liquid into bowls and serve with fresh crusty bread.

PUY LENTIL AND SPINACH SALAD

Serve this as a substantial side salad with sausages or baked fish. It contains nori, which in addition to valuable nutrients adds a tanginess that complements the earthy lentils. The seaweed is toasted first to improve its flavor, aroma, and texture.

preparation time 5 minutes
cooking time 30–35 minutes
serves 2

Contains fiber, protein, folate, vitamins B, C, E and K, calcium, manganese, iron, magnesium, phosphorus, potassium, copper

  2 tbsp olive oil
  1 small red onion, diced
  ½ red bell pepper, diced
  1 clove garlic, chopped
  1 cup Puy lentils, rinsed
  1 bay leaf
  1 tsp fresh thyme leaves
  2½ cups vegetable stock
  freshly squeezed lemon juice
  freshly ground black pepper
  1 sheet untoasted dried nori seaweed
  2 cups young spinach leaves, washed

• Heat the oil in a wide pan and cook the onion and red bell pepper until the onion is soft but not browned, about 5 minutes, adding the garlic 1 minute before the end.
• Add the lentils, bay leaf, and thyme, stirring until warmed through.
• Add enough stock to cover the lentils by about ½ inch and bring to a boil. Reduce the heat and simmer for 20–25 minutes, or until the lentils are tender, but retain a little bite.
• Season to taste with the lemon juice and black pepper.
• Toast the glossy, smooth side of the nori sheet very quickly over an open flame, until it becomes dark green, then sprinkle a little over the lentils.
• Serve with the spinach leaves.

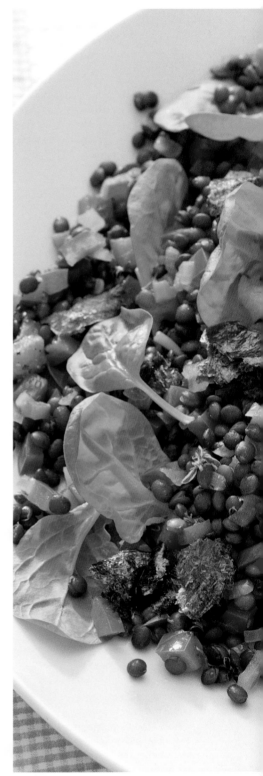

ROASTED AUTUMN VEGETABLES

This is hearty fare for the first cold nights of the year. Home-grown winter squash store well on a windowsill, so you can make this through the winter, too (when celeriac makes a tasty addition). Cut the sweet potato and carrots into equal-size 1 inch chunks. Seaweed salt transforms this dish.

preparation time 10 minutes
cooking time 40–50 minutes
serves 2

Contains fiber, protein, beta-carotene, folate, vitamins C and K, potassium, copper, manganese, selenium

1 small (or ½ large) butternut squash or home-grown pumpkin, quartered and seeded, then cut into wedges
1 sweet potato, peeled and cut into chunks
3 unpeeled onions, quartered
2 organic carrots, cut into chunks
2 uncooked beets, peeled and quartered
1 red bell pepper, halved and seeded
4 cloves garlic, peeled
olive oil, for drizzling
sea salt and freshly ground black pepper, to taste
4 sprigs of fresh rosemary
1 cup ready cooked and peeled whole chestnuts
6 slices bacon, cut into bite-size pieces
Worcestershire or soy sauce, to taste

• Preheat the oven to 300°F.
• In a sheet pan, place the squash, sweet potato, onions, carrot, beet, red bell pepper, and garlic. Drizzle with olive oil and sprinkle with sea salt then put in the oven to roast.
• After 20 minutes add the rosemary, chestnuts, and bacon. Check the pan to see whether any of the vegetables are tender to the touch and transfer those that are ready to a large serving dish and keep warm. The sweet potato, garlic, beet, and pepper will be done in 20–30 minutes.
• After 40 minutes' cooking time, check that the rest of the vegetables are soft and caramelized. Any not quite done can be left in the oven for up to 10 minutes more.
• Turn everything out into the serving dish and mix well, removing the papery onion skins.
• Season with black pepper, a little sea salt, and a few dashes of Worcestershire (or soy) sauce.

BEET SALAD

Rich in color and robust in flavor, this no-cook root-vegetable salad is palate-cleansing, and good served with oily fish. Do wear an apron when preparing this one: beet juice stains.

preparation time 5 minutes
cooking time 0
serves 2

Contains fiber, beta-carotene, folate, vitamins C and K, potassium, manganese

4 organic carrots
2 uncooked beets
generous handful of sunflower seeds
balsamic vinegar, to taste

• Top and tail the carrots and peel the beets. Shred all the vegetables and transfer to a bowl.
• Toast the sunflower seeds in a dry skillet, and toss into the shredded carrots and beets while still warm.
• Dress with a little balsamic vinegar, toss well and serve immediately.

HARVEST CRUMBLE

Much of the bounty for this dessert is free for the picking from the autumn hedgerow—blackberries, hazelnuts, and even apples. For maximum nutrients, substitute the fruit with whatever variety is most ripe this week in your region.

preparation time 10–15 minutes
cooking time 30 minutes
serves 4

Contains fiber, manganese, magnesium, phosphorus, selenium, vitamin E, zinc

3 cups blackberries
1½ cups peeled, cored, and sliced apples
2 tbsp brown sugar
7 tablespoons cold butter
¾ cup whole-wheat flour
¾ cup jumbo oats
¼ cup hazelnuts, crushed with a pestle
3 tbsp pumpkin seeds
Sour cream, Greek yogurt, or clotted cream, to serve

• Preheat the oven to 375°F.
• Place the blackberries and apple slices at the bottom of a pie dish. Sprinkle over 1 tbsp of the sugar.
• Place the flour in a bowl. Cut the butter into pieces and blend into the flour until the mixture resembles coarse bread crumbs.
• Stir in the oats, hazelnut pieces, seeds, and the remaining sugar. Moisten with 2 tsp water.
• Pile the crumble topping over the fruit and bake for 30 minutes, or until lightly browned on top.
• Serve with sour cream, Greek yogurt or, for a treat, clotted cream.

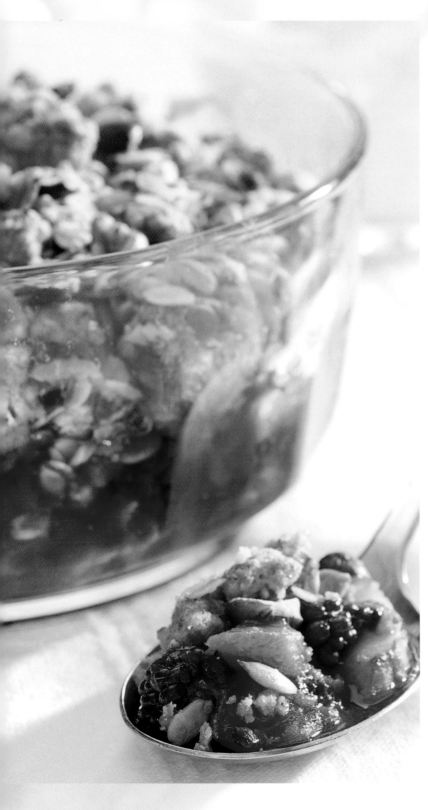

BAKED APPLES

This makes an incredibly comforting pudding that takes just minutes to prepare. Serve with homemade custard or good-quality organic vanilla ice cream.

preparation time 5 minutes
cooking time 45–50 minutes
serves 2

Contains fiber, manganese, vitamin E, copper

2 large cooking apples
2 tbsp apple juice, for steaming
⅓ cup sliced almonds
3 tbsp hazelnuts, cut into pieces
1 tbsp raisins
4 dried figs, chopped
¼ cup firmly packed brown sugar
½ tsp ground cinnamon
2 tbsp butter

• Preheat the oven to 375°F.
• Core the apples, either with an apple corer or a sharp knife, leaving the apple in one piece. Score around the "waist" of each apple.
• Place the apples in a deep, ovenproof dish, with a little apple juice in the bottom.
• Toast the nuts in a dry skillet over low heat, then place in a bowl with the raisins, chopped figs, sugar, and cinnamon. Mix well to combine.
• Spoon the fruit and nut mixture into the cavities of the apples, squashing it down well, and top each apple with 1 tbsp butter.
• Bake the apples for 45 minutes, or until they are soft enough that a knife slides easily into the flesh.
• Serve immediately.

WINTER WARMERS

EGGS FLORENTINE

A breakfast classic and just the thing to start a winter weekend or indulgent brunch. Serve with a floury muffin. This version uses whole-wheat flour and olive oil for a nuttier taste. For another twist on the original, substitute kale for spinach—just chop it extra fine. Kale retains some crunchiness, while spinach wilts.

preparation time 5 minutes
cooking time 15 minutes
serves 2

Contains fiber, protein, calcium, beta-carotene, vitamins B_6, C and K, calcium, potassium, copper, manganese, selenium, phosphorus

2 tbsp olive oil
1/4 cup whole-wheat flour
2/3 cup organic milk
2/3 cup shredded sharp cheddar cheese
2 tsp Dijon mustard
5 cups spinach or kale, washed and tough stems removed
4 eggs
1 tsp vinegar (optional)
sea salt and freshly ground black pepper
2 English muffins
butter, to serve

• First make a cheese sauce: heat the olive oil in a pan and stir in the flour, allowing it to cook gently for 1 minute.
• Add the milk little by little, stirring constantly to prevent lumps. Once you have a sauce thick enough to coat the back of a spoon (you may not need all the milk), stir in the cheese and the mustard. Beat until smooth, then cover and set aside in a warm place.
• Place the spinach or kale leaves in a

pan with the washing water clinging to the leaves and put on the lid. Allow to steam until the leaves wilt, about 1 minute (or longer for kale). Strain, then cover and set aside in a warm place.
• Poach the eggs: either use a poacher or, one at a time, crack each into a cup and slide into a pan of boiling water containing 1 tsp vinegar (optional). For safety's sake, poach until the yolk is hard, about 5 minutes.
• To serve, arrange 1/2 the leaves as a "bed" on each plate, top with 2 eggs, pour over 1/2 the cheese sauce, and season with sea salt and pepper.
• Toast the muffins, then butter and serve on the side.

JERUSALEM ARTICHOKE SOUP

This simple, velvet-textured soup has a rich earthiness that goes well with toasted sourdough bread. Don't tell others the main ingredient of this soup—keep them guessing before showing them one of the knobbly tubers.

preparation time 5 minutes
cooking time 35 minutes
serves 2

Contains fiber, iron, vitamin C, folate, potassium, phosphorus, magnesium, copper

1 1/4 lb Jerusalem artichokes, scrubbed well
juice of 1 lemon
2 tbsp olive oil
1 onion, chopped
2 celery sticks, chopped
2 cloves garlic, chopped
4 cups vegetable stock

sea salt and freshly ground black pepper
1 tbsp chopped fresh parsley leaves
sour cream, to serve

• Slice the artichokes roughly (no need to peel if they are very well scrubbed) and drop into a bowl containing half the lemon juice to prevent the flesh from discoloring.
• Pour the olive oil into a large pan, then sweat the onion and celery until the onion is soft but not colored.
• Drain the artichoke slices and add to a pan with the garlic; stir through for 5 minutes. Pour over enough of the stock to cover the artichokes plus the remaining lemon juice.
• Cover and allow to simmer over medium heat until the artichokes are soft, about 20–25 minutes. Let cool.
• Place the soup into a blender or food processor, reserving the pan, and whiz to your preferred consistency: some people like it smooth and others chunkier. If it seems a little thick, add a little boiling water and stir through. Season with salt and pepper, to taste, and reheat as necessary.
• Serve with a sprinkling of parsley and a swirl of sour cream.

PUMPKIN SOUP IN ITS OWN TUREEN

This is a stunning soup to serve at table. Do not use the large pumpkins intended for Halloween, which are not grown for eating; use a heavy culinary specialty, such as Tom Hubbard, that keeps well into winter. Choose a medium-size pumpkin; a large one may collapse in on itself. If this does happen, scrape everything into a blender and whiz to combine.

preparation time 10 minutes
cooking time 2 hours
serves 4

Contains fiber, beta-carotene, vitamins B_2, C and E, potassium, copper, manganese

1 medium pumpkin
2 tbsp olive oil
sea salt and freshly ground black pepper, to season
1 medium onion, chopped
1 tsp ground ginger
1 tsp ground cumin
4 cups hot vegetable or chicken stock
handful of hazelnuts, toasted, to garnish

• Preheat the oven to 375°F.
• Cut the top off the pumpkin to make a lid and scrape out the seeds and stringy bits (reserve the seeds to toast and eat as a snack with a little salt).
• Place the pumpkin in a deep, wide, ovenproof dish. Rub the olive oil and a little salt and pepper into the flesh.
• Place the chopped onion and the spices in the pumpkin, then pour in as much of the stock as required to fill the pumpkin. Replace the lid, cover with foil and bake for 1½–2 hours, depending on the size of the pumpkin and the thickness of the flesh.
• Halfway through the cooking time, scrape some of the flesh into the soup, but try not to dig too hard or the shell

may collapse. Repeat scraping the sides again at the end of the cooking time. The soup is ready when the flesh is so soft that it "melts" into the stock.
• Correct the seasoning and serve garnished with the hazelnuts.

COLESLAW

This crunchy red and green winter salad is a great source of folate and vitamins B and K. It's a great accompaniment to a wide range of dishes, such as baked potatoes and sausages.

preparation time 15 minutes
cooking time 0
serves 2

Contains fiber; calcium, beta-carotene, vitamins B, C, K and E, folate, potassium, manganese, magnesium, phosphorus, copper

½ red cabbage, washed
good handful of Swiss chard or spinach leaves, washed and stalks removed
1 large organic carrot, shredded
1 tart apple, peeled and shredded
handful of raisins
3–4 tbsp store-bought mayonnaise
freshly ground black pepper, to taste

• Thinly shred the cabbage and the chard or spinach leaves and pile into a large serving bowl.
• Mix in the shredded carrot and apple and the raisins.
• Stir in the mayonnaise well and season with pepper.

BROILED OYSTERS

There's not much to these winter delicacies, but each one is packed with protein and zinc, which is handy when you require maximum nutrition in a tiny bite. It's probably best to ask your fish merchant to shuck the oysters for you; this is much more effortful than the cooking. Ask him to keep the juice for you. Discard any oysters that look dry or smell unpleasant.

preparation time 10 minutes
cooking time 9 minutes
serves 2

Contains protein, calcium, vitamin B_{12}, iron, zinc, copper, magnesium, selenium

4 tbsp organic butter
1 shallot, very finely chopped
2 cloves garlic, very finely chopped
12 oysters, opened
½ cup grated Parmesan cheese
freshly ground black pepper
1 tbsp chopped fresh parsley leaves
lemon wedges, to serve

• Melt the butter in a pan, add the shallot and cook until soft but not colored. Add the garlic toward the end. Leave in a warm place to infuse.
• Preheat the broiler to a high heat.
• Place the opened oysters on heatproof serving plates with some of their juice and a sprinkling of Parmesan cheese. Spoon a little of the melted garlic-shallot butter over the top and a little pepper and parsley. You may not need all the butter and Parmesan.
• Place the dishes under the broiler until the cheese is brown and bubbling, around 2–3 minutes.
• Serve immediately, with lemon wedges.

SPINACH AND POTATO CURRY

Olive oil isn't the traditional Indian frying medium, but it doesn't detract from the flavor of this curry. This is not super hot, but if your palate is delicate, substitute paprika for the chili powder and serve with extra yogurt. Serve on top of basmati rice.

preparation time 10 minutes
cooking time 25 minutes
serves 2–3

Contains fiber, beta-carotene, vitamins B_6, C and K, folate, calcium, iron, potassium, manganese, copper, magnesium

1 lb unpeeled potatoes, well scrubbed
sea salt, to taste
1 tsp coriander seeds
1 tbsp olive oil
1 medium onion, finely chopped
2 cloves garlic, finely chopped
1 inch fresh ginger root, peeled and chopped
1 tsp ground turmeric
½ tsp chili powder
1 lb spinach, well washed and finely chopped
½ teaspoon garam masala
yogurt, for serving
1 tbsp chopped fresh cilantro leaves

• Bring the potatoes to a boil in lightly salted water for 10 minutes, until they are still firm but soft enough to stick in a knife. Drain and set aside.
• While the potatoes are boiling, grind the coriander seeds to a fine powder using a mortar and pestle.
• In a large pan, lightly cook the onion with the garlic and ginger. When the onion is just turning brown, add a little salt, the turmeric, chili powder, and ground coriander.
• Cut the parboiled potatoes into small chunks and add to the mixture in the pan, frying gently until the potatoes are almost soft, about 10 minutes.
• Put the spinach leaves with the washing water still clinging to the leaves into the pan. Cook for several minutes until the spinach has wilted and everything is nicely blended.
• Just before serving, stir through the garam masala.
• Serve with plenty of yogurt and garnished with the chopped cilantro leaves.

SAVOY CABBAGE AND RED PEPPER PASTA

The flavor of Savoy cabbage marries well with red bell pepper, pine nuts, and Parmesan. Do use the dark outer cabbage leaves—the darker the color, the more nutrients—but wash thoroughly.

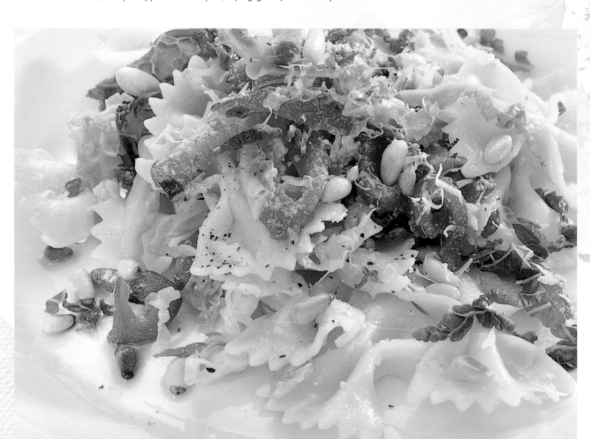

preparation time 15 minutes
cooking time 12–15 minutes
serves 2

Contains fiber, protein, beta-carotene, folate, vitamins B_6 and C, calcium, magnesium, potassium, manganese

1 red bell pepper
2 tbsp pine nuts
8 oz farfalle or other flat pasta
sea salt and freshly ground black pepper, to taste
extra-virgin olive oil, for drizzling
½ Savoy cabbage, finely shredded
1 cup grated Parmesan cheese, plus extra for serving

• Preheat the broiler and bring a pan of lightly salted water to a boil.
• Cut the pepper in half, pull out the seeds and place under the broiler, rounded sides facing upward, until the skins blacken and blister.
• Wrap the charred pepper halves in a clean dish towel for 10 minutes, then peel off and discard the skin and chop the flesh. Set aside.
• Dry-fry the pine nuts in a skillet until golden, turning to toast both sides, and set aside.
• Drop the pasta into the pan of boiling water and cook uncovered at a rolling boil, stirring occasionally to separate the pasta until just *al dente* (for timing, see pack instructions).
• Drain the pasta, reserving a little of the cooking water, and return the pasta to the pan over a gentle heat.
• Drizzle over some olive oil, then add the shredded cabbage and stir through until the cabbage is just wilted.
• Add the pepper slices and Parmesan, and a little of the cooking water if the ingredients seem a little sticky.
• Add the pine nuts and serve immediately, with black pepper and extra Parmesan at table.

PURPLE-SPROUTING BROCCOLI STIR-FRY

Once you try purple-sprouting, you'll find regular broccoli—or calabrese—fibrous and tasteless. If you can bear not eating the stalks lightly steamed—when they are as good as asparagus—try cooking them in a stir-fry. Substitute seasonal vegetables through the winter for the ones listed here. Cut everything into fine julienne strips. Serve with boiled rice or egg noodles.

preparation time 10 minutes
cooking time 5 minutes
serves 2

Contains fiber, beta-carotene, vitamins B_2 and B_6, C, E and K, folate, potassium, manganese, magnesium

2 tbsp walnut oil
1 carrot, very finely sliced
½ small onion, finely chopped
1 tbsp freshly grated ginger root
2 cloves garlic, finely chopped
1 star anise
1 green bell pepper, seeded and sliced
⅓ cup almonds
8 oz purple-sprouting broccoli, with leaves
1 tbsp fish sauce (nam pla)
1 tbsp soy sauce
1 tbsp sesame seeds

• Heat the oil in a wok or large pan, then stir in the carrot, onion, ginger, garlic, and star anise and cook over high heat until fragrant, 1–2 minutes.
• Add the pepper, almonds, purple-sprouting broccoli, and fish and soy sauce, keeping all the ingredients moving around the pan for 2–3 minutes, or until the purple-sprouting broccoli is just soft.
• Just before serving, stir in the sesame seeds.

RICE PUDDING

This dish is so comforting in winter; what's more, it's a doddle to make. Older babies and toddlers love it, too. The rice doesn't look like nearly enough at the start, but don't be tempted to add more. Serve with sour cream for extra creaminess.

preparation time 5 minutes
cooking time around 2 hours
serves 4

Contains protein, fiber, vitamins B_2 and B_{12}, D, E and K, calcium, phosphorus

2 tablespoons cold organic butter, plus extra for greasing
4 cups whole organic milk
½ cup short-grain (pudding) rice
½ tsp vanilla extract
3 tbsp sugar
handful of pitted prunes
1 nutmeg
2 tbsp sliced almonds

• Preheat the oven to 300°F. Butter a large ovenproof bowl or casserole dish and place the rice in it.
• Heat the milk to simmering point in a pan and pour over the rice. Stir in the vanilla extract, sugar, and prunes.
• Dot the top with pieces of cold butter and grate a good sprinkling of nutmeg over the top.
• Place in the oven, uncovered, for 2 hours, or until golden brown on top.
• Toward the end of the cooking time, toast the almonds in a dry pan until golden, then sprinkle over each portion as you serve it.

winter warmers

111

SPRING DELIGHTS

FAVA BEAN DIP

This makes a lovely, bright green dip. Use the most tender beans—skin and all. At the start of the season, just show the beans the water. Toward the end of the season, you will need to cook them for a little longer. Serve with pita or flat bread and crudités.

preparation time 15 minutes
cooking time 20 minutes
serves 2

Contains fiber, protein, folate, calcium, iron

2 cups shelled fava beans
2 cloves garlic, coarsely chopped
4 scallions, coarsely chopped
½ tsp ground cumin
1 tbsp sour cream
juice of ½ lemon
sea salt and freshly ground black pepper
dillweed, to garnish

• Blanch the fava beans in a little water until just soft; drain, reserving the cooking water.
• Once cool enough to handle, slip the skins off the beans and discard.
• Place the beans in a blender or food processor with the garlic, scallions, cumin, and the sour cream and whiz until smooth.
• Add the lemon juice, then season to taste with sea salt and pepper. If the dip is too thick, add a little of the cooking water.
• Serve garnished with fronds of dillweed.

BROCCOLI SOUP

Eat this soup regularly through pregnancy and when breastfeeding to prime your baby to enjoy the acquired bitterness of broccoli. It should seem familiar and enjoyable to your baby when you start giving solids.

preparation time 5 minutes
cooking time 15 minutes
serves 2

Contains fiber, beta-carotene, vitamins C, E and K, folate, potassium, manganese, calcium

1 tbsp olive oil
1 medium onion, chopped
1 head of broccoli (calabrese), about 10 oz
2½ cups ml vegetable stock
freshly ground black pepper, to season
2 tbsp Greek yogurt

• In a large pan, heat the oil and sweat the onion.
• Meanwhile, cut through the broccoli stem about 1 inch below the head.
• When the onion is soft add 2 inches in height of stock to the pan and stand the broccoli head in it. Carefully pour in more stock so the florets stand just above the stock. Put on the lid and simmer for 5–10 minutes, or until the florets are soft, but still bright green. Do not overcook. Let cool and reserve pan.
• Place the soup in a blender or food processor and whiz to a smooth consistency, adding more stock or water if the soup seems thick or grainy.
• Reheat as required then season with pepper. Stir a swirl of Greek yogurt into each bowl just before serving.

FRESH PEA FRITTATA

This very sweet, Italian-inspired omelet is good if you have a glut of fresh peas. Peas are the richest source of vitamin B_1, and fresh peas have been shown to enhance sleep, raise a jaded appetite, and boost cheerfulness. Accompany with a green or tomato salad.

preparation time 10 minutes
cooking time 15–20 minutes
serves 2–3

Contains protein, vitamins B, C and K, selenium, manganese, choline, folate

2 tbsp olive oil
2 tbsp fresh shredded mint leaves
1⅓ cups shelled fresh peas
3 large, free range eggs
¼ cup grated Parmesan cheese
salt and freshly ground black pepper

• Preheat the broiler to moderate. Heat the oil in a heavy, ovenproof skillet over low-to-medium heat.
• Add the mint and peas and warm through, stirring until *al dente*, about 3–5 minutes.
• Beat the eggs in a bowl with the Parmesan, season, then pour over the peas, tipping the pan so the egg is well distributed (it may not look as though there is enough egg).
• Cook for 5–10 minutes, or until the egg has set around the edges. It should still be gooey on top.
• Place under the broiler until the top is just set and golden (but not brown or crispy), about 3 minutes.
• Slide a knife or spatula around the edge to loosen the frittata, then place a plate on top and invert to transfer to the plate—it may need a little help.
• When cool, slice and serve.

SOURDOUGH BREAD

Kneading bread is a very calming, meditative action if you're feeling stressed or preoccupied by the many worries of pregnancy. Sourdough makes the minerals in the flour more available for the body to absorb; it also makes great toast. Begin this recipe before going to bed, leaving it to rise overnight.

preparation time (including rising time) up to 24 hours
cooking time 35–40 minutes
makes 1 large loaf

Contains protein, fiber, folate, B vitamins, lactobacillus

3 cups strong white organic bread flour
⅔ cup whole-wheat organic flour
3 tsp salt
1–1¼ cups sourdough starter (see page 100)
1 cup boiling water
2 tsp raw honey

• Place the flours and salt in a large mixing bowl.
• Make a well in the center and pour in the starter. Draw in flour from the side of the bowl little by little, then add the water and stir into a sticky mass.
• Tip onto a floured board and knead by pushing, pulling, folding, and turning—adding flour to your hands and the board as necessary to keep the dough from sticking. Work for at least 10 minutes, until the dough is springy and silky smooth.
• Place the dough in a clean, oiled bowl, turn to coat in the oil, cover with a dish towel and leave at room temperature overnight, or until doubled in size (it will take longer if the room is cool).
• Replenish the starter by feeding it (see page 100).
• Next morning, or when the dough

has doubled in size (the longer it takes, the better the tangy flavor), knock the dough back by punching it to deflate it, then return to the oiled bowl and cover with a clean dish towel again.
• Allow to double in size again (this may take all day).
• Preheat the oven to 390°F with a baking sheet inside.
• Remove the baking sheet, dust with flour and invert the bowl of dough onto the sheet. Slash the top with a sharp knife.
• Mist the inside of the oven with water using a plant spray, then quickly put in the loaf.
• Bake for 15 minutes, then reduce the heat to 350°F for another 20–25 minutes, or until the loaf is golden brown and sounds hollow when tapped on the bottom.
• Allow to cool on a wire rack.

SMOKED MACKEREL SALAD

Late spring sees the start of the mackerel season. These oily fish are one of the best sources of omega-3 fatty acids, which form the building blocks of your baby's developing nervous system and brain. This is an easy salad to throw together from ingredients in the refrigerator.

preparation time 10 minutes
cooking time 13 minutes
serves 2–3

Contains omega-3 fatty acids, protein, folate, vitamins C and K, selenium

1½ lb unpeeled new or salad potatoes, left whole or cut in half if large
1 whole or 2 fillets smoked mackerel
½ cup cherry tomatoes, cut in half
½ yellow bell pepper, diced
½ red bell pepper, diced
½ bunch scallions, chopped (including the green)

1 bunch asparagus or 3½ oz purple-sprouting broccoli
2 tsp balsamic vinegar
3 tbsp extra-virgin olive oil
½ lemon
1 tsp Dijon mustard
1 tsp honey
sea salt and freshly ground black pepper, to taste

• Bring the potatoes to a boil and simmer until just tender, about 10 minutes. While they are cooking, cut the fish into bite-size pieces and place in a large serving bowl with the tomatoes, chunks of pepper, and scallions.
• Drain the potatoes, reserving the cooking water and bringing it back to a simmer. Toss the potatoes with the fish and vegetables in the bowl.
• Slice the asparagus, if using, discarding the woody ends, and add the pieces of asparagus or purple-sprouting broccoli to the boiling water until just soft, about 2–3 minutes.
• Drain and place in the bowl with the other ingredients.
• Beat together the balsamic vinegar, oil, squeeze of lemon juice, mustard, honey, and seasoning.
• Pour over the salad and toss to coat, then serve immediately.

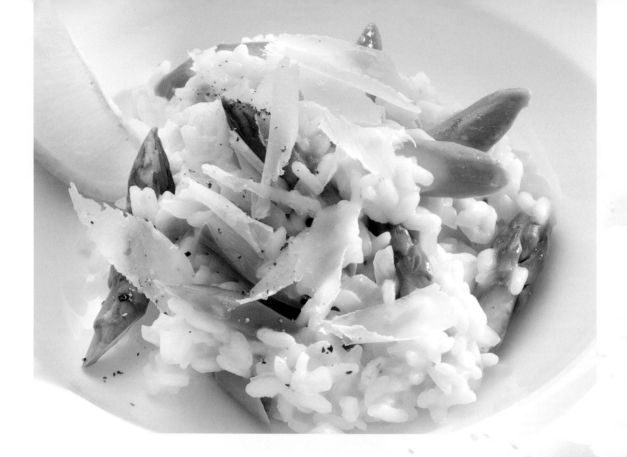

RISOTTO WITH ASPARAGUS AND PARMESAN

The act of stirring a risotto can feel quite meditative. Enjoy switching off and focus your thoughts on your baby as you stir. If you use brown risotto rice, allow at least 40 minutes longer for the dish to cook after you start adding stock. If you run out of stock and the rice is still hard, add boiled water.

preparation time 5 minutes
cooking time 30–40 minutes
serves 2

Contains fiber, protein, vitamins C, E and K, beta-carotene, B vitamins, folate, iron, phosphorus, potassium, copper, manganese, selenium

1 bunch asparagus
3⅓ cups chicken stock
3 tbsp olive oil
1 small onion, finely chopped
1½ cups risotto rice (carnaroli or arborio)
½ cup white wine
sea salt and freshly ground black pepper, to taste
4 tablespoons butter
¾ cup grated Parmesan plus extra for serving
1 lemon

• Cut off the woody ends of the asparagus, then slice the stems into about ½ inch lengths, leaving the tips intact (set the tips to one side).
• Bring the stock to a boil and keep it on a low simmer.
• In a large pan heat the oil and cook the onion until soft, but not coloured.
• Add the rice and the chopped asparagus stems, stirring continuously

until the rice is golden, then pour in the wine—it will sizzle (don't worry, the alcohol burns off).
• Stir until the wine has evaporated, then add a ladleful of stock and lower the heat.
• Once the first ladleful of stock has been absorbed, add another—you should hear the pan "gasp" as you add more stock. Repeat, stirring constantly, for 20–30 minutes. Wait until you see a half-moon shape made by the spoon in the bottom of the pan before adding another ladleful. You may not need all the stock.
• After you have added half the stock, stir in the asparagus tips.
• Once the rice is soft and creamy but still has a little "bite," check and adjust the seasoning, turn off the heat, add the butter and Parmesan, cover and leave while the flavors absorb.
• Serve the risotto with a good squeeze of lemon juice.

RABBIT IN A POT

Much more nutritionally dense than a supermarket chicken, rabbit is one of the healthiest meats to eat during pregnancy. If unavailable at your local butcher's, try an organic meat delivery company. If squeamish, request a ready-jointed rabbit.

preparation time 15 minutes
cooking time 1 hour 40 minutes
serves 2–3

Contains omega-3 fatty acids, protein, folate, vitamins C and K, selenium

whole-wheat flour, seasoned, for
dusting
1 rabbit, jointed
2–4 tbsp olive oil
2 large onions, coarsely chopped
4 celery sticks, coarsely chopped
2 large carrots, coarsely chopped
4 bay leaves
2 cups chicken stock
⅔ cup dried porcini
sea salt and freshly ground black
pepper, to taste
1 tbsp chopped chives

• Preheat the oven to 300°F.
• Put the seasoned flour on a plate and roll the rabbit joints in it until coated.
• Heat the oil in a skillet and brown the joints on both sides, then transfer to a casserole.
• Add the onion and cook until soft but not colored. Add to the casserole with the other chopped vegetables and bay leaves.
• Pour over the chicken stock, add the porcini, season to taste, and top up with hot water, if necessary, to just cover the meat.
• Bring to a simmer, put on a lid and transfer to the oven for 1½ hours, or until the meat is tender (wild rabbit will take longer than farmed).
• Serve the rabbit sprinkled with the chives and with mashed potato and wilted spinach.

STEAK AU POIVRE

Steak is a common lust-after food during pregnancy and this is a delicious way to eat it. The steak can be prepared several hours ahead. If you are extra sensitive to heat right now, just reduce the amount of peppercorns.

preparation time 10 minutes
cooking time 13 minutes
serves 2–3

Contains protein, vitamin B$_{12}$, iron, zinc, selenium

1 tbsp black peppercorns, crushed
2 tbsp olive oil
2 large cloves garlic, crushed
2 sirloin steaks
⅔ cup sour cream
1 tsp tarragon
½ tsp dry mustard
2 tbsp brandy
salt, to season

• Place the peppercorns in a wide dish with the olive oil and garlic and stir to combine.
• Flatten the steaks with a meat mallet or rolling pin and place them side-by-side in the dish, turning so that each side is well coated with the peppery garlic oil. Cover and refrigerate for at least an hour.
• Mix together the sour cream, mustard powder, and tarragon in a small bowl.
• Heat a heavy skillet until very hot, then place the steaks in the pan; sear them for 1 minute on each side.
• Lower the heat and then cook the steaks for up to another 5 minutes (for well-done), turning halfway through. Serve onto a plate to rest.
• Pour the brandy into the pan and let it bubble and reduce (don't worry, this gets rid of the alcohol). Add the sour cream mixture, stirring it into the brandy-peppercorn juices and allowing it to reduce until slightly thicker. Stir in

any meat juices from the resting steaks. Taste and add a little salt, if necessary.
• Spoon the sauce over the steaks and serve with a watercress salad and chunky fries or boiled new potatoes.

LEMON CURD

With all the goodness of lemons and eggs, this preserve makes a creamy filling for a lemon tart or is delicious spread on toast. You will need sterilized glass jars with lids still hot from the oven or dishwasher, plus waxed disks.

preparation time 40 minutes
cooking time 15 minutes
makes 2 jars

Contains protein, B vitamins, folate, potassium, choline, vitamin C

4 unwaxed organic lemons
4 eggs
scant 1 cup superfine sugar
1 stick plus 1 tbsp unsalted butter

• Place the lemons in a warm place for 30 minutes, then roll them beneath your palm on a cutting board to maximize the juice.
• Zest the skin then juice the lemons.
• Beat the eggs with the sugar. Melt the butter in a heatproof bowl over a pan of simmering water, then beat in the egg and sugar mixture and the lemon zest and juice. Keep beating until the mixture thickens, about 8–10 minutes. Remove the mixture from the heat and spoon into the hot jars, filling them almost to the top. Put a wax disk on top of each jar and seal.
• Once cool, store in the refrigerator.

SUMMER RICHES

MUESLI

Start the day well with this hearty muesli topped with yogurt and fresh summer fruit. The combination of oats, nuts, and seeds will help you to feel calm and stay alert. If you suffer from pregnancy constipation, before bed, place a handful of prunes in a bowl and cover with water. Add to your morning muesli with some of the soaking water.

preparation time 15 minutes
cooking time 0
makes enough for 2 weeks

Contains protein, fiber, manganese, magnesium, selenium, vitamins B and E, folate, omega-3 fatty acids

5 cups jumbo organic oats
⅔ cup walnut pieces
1 cup sliced almonds
1 cup pumpkin seeds
⅔ cup sunflower seeds
3 tbsp pine nuts
3 tbsp sesame seeds

• Pour the oats into a large jar with an airtight lid, then add as many of the nuts and seeds as suit your palate, stirring them in until well combined.
• Replace the lid and store in a cool, dark place.
• Each morning, spoon 3–4 tbsp into a bowl and pour over lowfat organic milk and 1–2 tbsp plain organic yogurt.
• Allow to soak for 5 minutes before adding more milk, as necessary.
• Top with summer berries and/or chunks of melon or soft fruit.

SUMMER BEAN SALAD

Make this easy no-cook salad ahead of serving—the longer it sits in the fragrant juices, the tastier it gets. For speed, use canned, ready-cooked beans. This makes enough for several meals and is good in lunch boxes; store in the refrigerator.

preparation time 10 minutes
cooking time 0
serves 4

Contains fiber, protein, vitamins C, A and K, potassium, manganese, folate

1 x 15 oz can kidney beans
1 x 15 oz can cranberry beans
1 x 15 oz can cannellini or lima beans
1 red bell pepper, diced
1 yellow bell pepper, diced
1 small red onion, chopped
4 sticks celery, chopped
1 cup cherry tomatoes, halved
1 tbsp chopped fresh parsley leaves
juice of 1 lemon
1–2 tbsp extra-virgin olive oil
sea salt and freshly ground black pepper, to taste

• Drain the beans, rinse, and put in a large serving bowl.
• Stir in the diced pepper, the onion and celery (add as much of the leafy fronds of celery as possible), and the halved tomatoes.
• Carefully mix in the herbs.
• Add enough lemon juice and olive oil to cover lightly, season, and toss.

HUMMUS

Homemade hummus is much tastier and cheaper than store-bought versions; using dried chickpeas really improves the taste. Serve with pita bread and crudités.

preparation time overnight soaking plus 2 hours simmering
cooking time 10 minutes
makes 8 large servings

Contains fiber, protein, iron, vitamin C, copper, folate, manganese

3 cups dried chickpeas
¾ cup tahini
6 cloves garlic, or to taste, chopped
2 tsp ground cumin
2 tsp ground coriander
1 tsp paprika (Spanish Pimenton Dulce is best)
zest and juice of 2 large, unwaxed organic lemons
¼ cup extra-virgin olive oil
sea salt and freshly ground black pepper, to season

• Soak the chickpeas overnight in plenty of water
• When ready to cook, change the water, bring to a boil and simmer, uncovered, for 2 hours. Do not salt the water, and skim off foam as it rises to the surface. When the chickpeas are soft but still have a little bite, drain them, reserving the cooking water.
• Whiz the chickpeas with the rest of the ingredients plus ½ cup of the cooking water in a blender or food processor. If too dry, add more water.
• Season to taste, adding a little more lemon juice, olive oil, or paprika as necessary, and whiz again to lighten the texture slightly.

AVOCADO GAZPACHO

The addition of avocados to this cooling but filling soup contributes extra protein to a summer staple. Make it with the ripest, tastiest ingredients you can find. Don't be put off by the baby food-like appearance!

preparation time 40 minutes
cooking time 0
serves 2–3

Contains vitamin C, beta-carotene, vitamin K, potassium, manganese, folate

2 oz stale artisan white bread
2 cloves garlic, chopped
2 tsp sea salt
6 large ripe tomatoes (Marmande are good), chopped
½ onion, chopped
½ cucumber, peeled and diced
½ green bell pepper, seeded and chopped
2 very ripe avocados
2 tbsp olive oil
1 tbsp white wine vinegar
juice of ½ lemon

To garnish
1 hard-cooked egg, diced
½ green bell pepper, seeded and diced
2 scallions, finely chopped

• Soak the bread in water for 30 minutes, until soft, then squeeze it out.
• Whiz using a blender or food processor with the garlic, salt, tomatoes, onion, cucumber, bell pepper, and the flesh from the avocados, until you have a rough-textured paste.
• Gradually add the olive oil, vinegar, and lemon juice and blend again, adding enough chilled water to make a soup-like consistency.
• Chill and serve cold, adding ice cubes, and garnish with the egg, bell pepper, and scallions.

TORTILLA

This is tastiest when eaten at room temperature, and as well as a light lunch is perfect picnic or lunchbox fare, when cut into slices. Accompany with a few olives, green beans, and a crisp salad.

preparation time 10 minutes
cooking time 30–40 minutes
serves 4

Contains vitamin C, beta-carotene, vitamin K, potassium, manganese, folate

4 large, waxy potatoes
¾ cup olive oil
1 medium onion, sliced
6 eggs
good pinch sea salt

• Cut the potatoes into 2½ inch slices, drop into a pan of water to rinse, then pat dry.
• Pour the oil into a large skillet over medium-hot heat; when hot, add the potato slices and cook with the onion over low-medium heat for 15 minutes, or until the potatoes are cooked but firm (don't let them brown). Drain into a colander, reserving the oil.
• While the potatoes are cooking, beat the eggs with the salt in a large bowl, then add the potato-onion mixture. Let it stand for 10 minutes.
• Place 2 tbsp of the reserved oil into a clean skillet over low-medium heat; when hot, pour in the egg-potato mixture and swirl it around so it floats free of the sides. Don't let it stick to the bottom. Cook until the bottom is set but the top is still somewhat runny, 5–10 minutes maximum.
• Place under a hot broiler to brown the top; don't cook until "dry," the residual heat will cook it through.

THREE-TOMATO SAUCE

This works best with the ripest of fresh tomatoes, but the canned and preserved tomatoes enrich the sauce if your home-grown produce is less than perfect. Serve with pasta and Parmesan cheese or over grilled fish or meatballs. Freeze leftovers for a taste of summer in midwinter.

preparation time 5 minutes
cooking time 25–30 minutes
serves 2–3

Contains vitamin C and K, beta-carotene, potassium, manganese, lycopene

2 tbsp extra-virgin olive oil
4 cloves garlic, finely sliced
3½ oz preserved tomatoes (see page 41)
1 x 14½ oz can whole plum tomatoes (Pelati or San Marzano)
1 tsp dried oregano
8 oz fresh ripe tomatoes, coarsely chopped
sea salt and freshly ground black pepper, to season

• Heat the oil in a heavy skillet over medium heat and briefly cook the garlic until fragrant but not browned, then stir in the preserved tomatoes until warmed through.
• Add the canned tomatoes, crushing each one between your fingers (leave the juice in the can for the time being) and the oregano. Simmer until reduced and thickened, about 15 minutes.
• Add the fresh tomatoes and allow to simmer until they have softened, about 10 minutes. Add some of the juice from the can if the sauce becomes too dry.
• Season to taste and serve over the pasta of your choice.

CHICKEN STOCK

Make this after enjoying roast chicken, then use as a base for soups and risotto. For a quick and easy soup, strain the stock then add cooked rice and canned corn kernels, bring it back to a simmer and add some of the reserved chicken meat. Heat through for a few minutes then serve.

preparation time 10 minutes
cooking time about 21/2 hours
makes about 2 quarts

Contains protein, B vitamins

1 roast chicken carcass
4 cloves garlic
2 celery sticks, coarsely chopped
1 large organic carrot, coarsely chopped
1 leek, cleaned and coarsely chopped
1 onion, peeled and cut in half
1 tsp whole black peppercorns
2 bay leaves
2 sprigs fresh thyme
2 sprigs fresh rosemary

• Cut away any remaining meat from the chicken carcass and set aside for soup, sandwiches, or stir-fries.
• Place the carcass, plus any remaining skin, cooking juices, or gravy into a pan and cover with cold water (include the cooking water from any vegetables)— you will need just under 3 quarts.
• Add the garlic and the chopped celery, carrot and leek, the onion, peppercorns, and herbs.
• Bring to a boil, then simmer on a low heat for as long as you can, at least 90 minutes and up to 2 hours, skimming off the scum as it rises to the surface. The longer you simmer, the better the flavor.
• Strain through a strainer, discarding the bones and vegetables, and transfer to pitchers. Allow to cool, then refrigerate.
• Once it has become jelly-like, divide into portions to freeze.

FISH PIE

Containing salmon and anchovies, this pie offers all the goodness of omega-3 fatty acids, which are so essential for your baby's developing brain and nervous system. Serve with peas, green beans, or spinach.

preparation time 10 minutes
cooking time 1 hour
serves 4

Contains protein, calcium, omega-3 fatty acids, vitamins D and B, beta-carotene, magnesium, selenium, iodine, phosphorus, choline

2¼ lb starchy potatoes
butter, for coating
2 eggs
14 oz salmon fillets
10 oz smoked haddock fillets
2 bay leaves
1 medium carrot, very finely sliced
1 celery stick, chopped
1 small onion, peeled and studded with 6 cloves
2 cups organic milk
3½ oz raw shelled shrimp, defrosted
2 or 3 preserved anchovies, torn into pieces
2 tbsp olive oil
sea salt and freshly ground black pepper, to taste
1 cup shredded sharp cheddar cheese
2 tbsp sour cream
2 tsp Dijon mustard
zest of 1 unwaxed, organic lemon

• Cut the potatoes into quarters (or eighths if large) and place in a pan of boiling, salted water. Simmer until just cooked, about 10 minutes, then drain.
• Return to the pan with a generous pat of butter and replace the lid.
• Meanwhile, hard-cook the eggs (for 7 minutes) and leave in a pan of cold water to cool.
• Place the fish in a wide skillet with the bay leaves, carrot slices, chopped

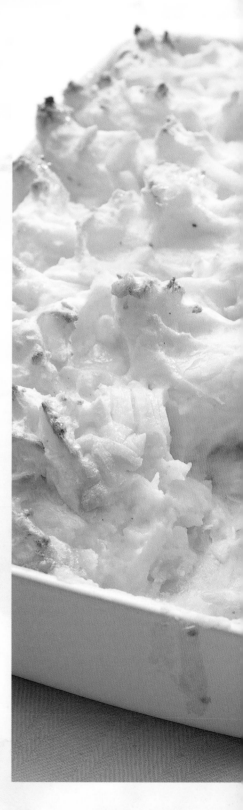

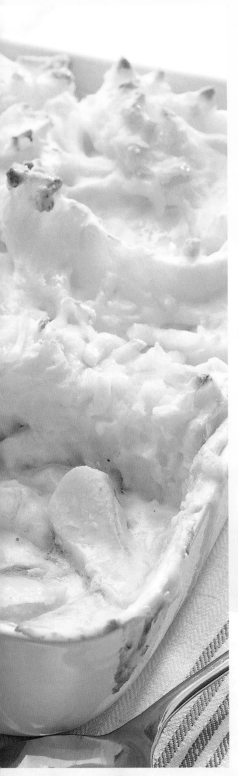

celery, and the clove-studded onion; cover with 1¾ cups of the milk. Bring to a simmer, then cook until the fish is cooked through, about 2–3 minutes.

• Scoop out the fish with a slotted spoon, leaving most of the carrots and celery in the milk, and transfer to an ovenproof baking dish, discarding any skin or bones. Reserve the milk and onion.

• Shell the eggs and quarter them. Add the shrimp, anchovy pieces, and quartered eggs to the fish, distributing them equally.

• Then mash the potatoes with the olive oil and a little of the remaining milk until fluffy, seasoning to taste.

• Preheat the oven to 350°F.

• Stir most of the cheese, the sour cream, and mustard into the reserved cooking milk with the lemon zest and bring to a simmer, beating until reduced a little, then pour over the fish mixture (discard the onion).

• Top with mashed potato and sprinkle the remaining grated cheese over the top. Bake for 25–30 minutes, until bubbling and brown on top.

SUMMER PUDDING

This is an incredibly easy, great-tasting pudding. Choose the fruit according to what's in the garden or hedgerow, altering the mix throughout the summer. Serve with Greek yogurt. If you're craving an instant berry hit, whiz up the fruit with a large pot of yogurt and a little Demerara sugar and serve as a fool.

preparation time overnight
cooking time 10 minutes
serves 4–6

Contains fiber, vitamins C and K, manganese, potassium

butter, for greasing
small loaf stale white bread (artisan, not supermarket white), thickly sliced with crusts removed
5 cups assorted dark-colored berries, currants or stoned fruit: blackberries, blueberries, raspberries, red or black currants, pitted damsons, or plums
¼–⅔ cup caster sugar (according to taste and the tartness of the fruit)

• Butter a large (4 cup) pudding bowl and line with the bread slices. First cut a piece to fit the bottom of the bowl, then build up the sides with wedge-shaped slices, making sure there are no gaps between them. Reserve enough bread for the top.

• Top and tail the fruit if necessary, then add to a large pan. Bring to a boil slowly with 1–2 tbsp water, then simmer until the fruit has broken down, less than 5 minutes.

• Taste and add sugar to taste (the pudding should be slightly tart).

• Pour the hot fruit with all the juices into the bowl, making sure it reaches almost to the top.

• Cover with bread, then place a saucer over the top. It must be small enough to sit neatly inside the rim of the bowl.

• Stand the bowl on a large plate, then weight down the saucer (old-fashioned weights from scales are ideal, or use full cans). Allow to cool, then refrigerate overnight.

• When ready to serve, remove the weights, run a knife around the inside of the bowl, then turn upside down onto a serving plate. If there are patches of white bread, smear juice over.

• Cut the pudding into thick wedges and serve with cream, sour cream, or Greek yogurt.

SAFETY ESSENTIALS

Pregnancy is a great excuse to take a little more care of yourself, whether by making sure that you don't skip breakfast or ensuring you cut down on strenuous work in the garden. You now have every excuse for relaxing with your feet up reading this book or leafing through seed catalogues, but in order to buy and grow the best possible food, there will be some risk-inherent practices that need adjusting, such as unavoidable carrying and, possibly, a little digging. Here's some vital information about staying safe—items to avoid, for example—and ways to make sure that you safeguard both your health and that of your baby.

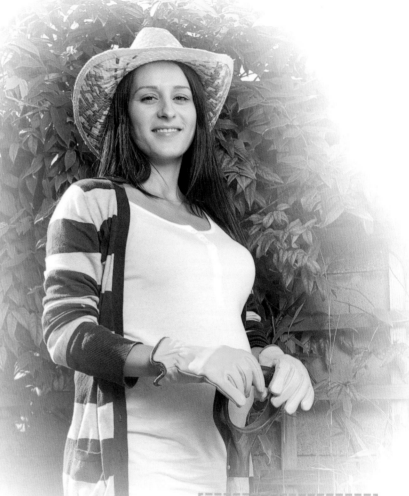

SAFE DRINKING AND EATING

Whether or not you are working outside or simply going about your daily routine, it is important to keep hydrated. An adequate fluid intake is essential during pregnancy to help your blood volume to increase and to supply your baby with nutrients. Also, because your body temperature is elevated during pregnancy, it's easier now to become dehydrated. Aim to drink at least 8 cups of fluids every day, the majority of which should be water. Milk and fruit and vegetable juices are also good but take care with herbal teas, caffeinated beverages, and alcohol.

FLUIDS TO AVOID

In moderate to large amounts, caffeine has been found to correlate with an increased risk of miscarriage. It can interfere with the absorption of folic acid and iron and can also lead to headaches and insomnia. Stick to less than 200 mg a day (1–2 cups of coffee, 2 cups of black tea or cocoa, 5 cans of cola, or 2 caffeine-containing energy drinks).

Green tea has been linked with depressing folic acid levels in the body and contains oxalic acid, which restricts calcium and iron absorption. It is best avoided before and during the first trimester.

Most experts agree that it is advisable to stop drinking alcohol completely while you are pregnant. On special occasions, however, you might have 1 glass of wine or beer, but don't do this more than once or twice a week and keep to standard

TAKE CARE

Avoid the following herbs commonly used in teas: ginseng, sage, rosemary, chamomile, hibiscus, lemongrass, parsley, valerian, fennel, licorice.

Before taking any other herbs medicinally, consult a herbalist who specializes in pregnancy.

strengths and bar measures.

There's lots of controversy about herbal teas in pregnancy. Herbalists value them for their medicinal properties, but many herbs commonly used in teas are uterine stimulants. If you decide to drink them, stick to a couple of cups a day and vary the type: ginger and tilleul, rosehip and the occasional peppermint tea may be considered safe by some medical practitioners. Choose organic teabags made by reputable companies, and don't brew your own from garden herbs.

PROBLEMATIC FOODS

Because of the risk of built-up teratogenic (fetus-harming) toxins in oily fish, such as mercury and PCBs (polychlorinated biphenyls), it is recommended that you eat no more than two portions a week while pregnant, trying for a baby, or breastfeeding. Eat a variety of fish rather than just one type—mackerel, sardines, salmon, trout, sea bream, sea bass, turbot, halibut, rock salmon, brown crabmeat—and avoid large fish such as shark, marlin, and swordfish, which are likely to be more contaminated. Do not have more than 2 tuna steaks or 4 cans of tuna a week.

Make sure, too, that you don't eat raw fish and raw shellfish, which can harbour bacteria including salmonella. Cooking to more than 145°F destroys the bacteria. Raw and soft-cooked eggs may also be contaminated with salmonella bacteria. Although it is unlikely to harm your baby, salmonella poisoning can make you very ill.

Meat served "rare," such as steak, cured meat like prosciutto, and products made from ground meat, such as burgers, may be infected

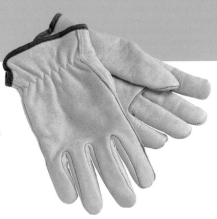

with the parasite toxoplasmosis, which can damage a baby's developing brain and eyes. Make sure all the meat you eat is very well cooked, with no pink remaining.

Pâtés that have not been pasteurized or UHT-treated may contain the listeria bug, as can "raw" milk cheeses (check the label), blue-veined cheese, and soft cheeses with a white rind—Brie, Camembert, and mold-ripened goat cheeses. In a tiny number of cases listeria can cause miscarriage or stillbirth.

INAPPROPRIATE NUTRIENTS

Too much retinol can harm your developing fetus, raising the risk of birth defects. For this reason avoid eating liver and liver pâté during pregnancy, which is too high in retinol to be safe. Also be sure to avoid fish-oil supplements and vitamin pills containing vitamin A for the same reason.

One study in 2009 linked a high intake of vitamin E with a heightened risk of congenital heart defects in newborns. However there are currently no recommendations on safe levels in pregnancy.

A Western diet typically consists of an unhealthy ratio of omega-6 to omega-3 fatty acids. To maximize the effect of the omega-3 fatty acids in your diet (see page 11), try to cut back on food containing omega-6 oils, which means anything containing sunflower, soy, corn, safflower, and canola oil—which means most store-bought cookies, cakes, pies, and savory snacks.

PROTECT YOURSELF

Wear rubber gloves at all times when gardening so you don't come into contact with chemicals in the soil and with cat toilet areas and animal feces, which may be infected with toxoplasmosis. If you find rubber gloves too heavy or hot, put on a pair of surgical gloves beneath your regular cotton gardening gloves. Deal with cuts and nicks as soon as you can, and wash your hands very well after gardening and before handling food.

Your skin will be more susceptible to the effects of sun now, due to the action of pregnancy hormones, so wear a sunscreen when working outdoors and a large-brimmed hat.

GO ORGANIC

It's important not to expose yourself to pesticides during pregnancy, especially in the first trimester, when you risk harming your baby's developing nervous system. This means avoiding everything you might currently be using to kill ants, wasps, slugs, weeds, or moss.

Now's the time to become weed tolerant and to use age-old deterrents, such as coffee grounds around young plants, mugs of beer set into the soil to catch slugs and a mild dish-washing liquid solution to spray aphid infestations.

If you are building raised beds, favor dense hardwood that doesn't need treatment, or eco-wood treated with borax or linseed. Avoid old timbers treated with creosote.

protect yourself

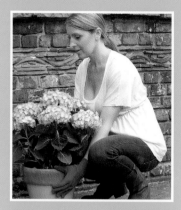

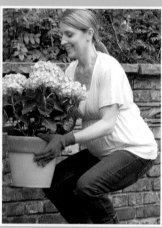

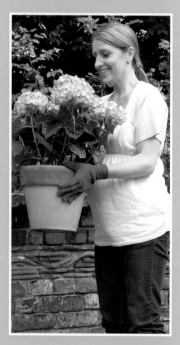

SAFE LIFTING AND CARRYING

During pregnancy, the ligaments and tendons that hold your joints securely in place become more elastic—that's to help you get the baby out!—so you have to be careful when exerting yourself; you simply won't be as stable as before pregnancy, and are more prone to soft-tissue injuries. Then there's the inconvenience of that bump, throwing your center of gravity out of balance. This can be a real issue when lifting and carrying, whether while out shopping or in the garden.

The key to safe lifting is to use the muscles in your legs rather than relying on your back and abdomen, and to move in a slow, controlled way—don't be tempted to use momentum to jerk up and down.

1 Stand directly in front of the item you wish to lift with feet hip-width apart and pointing forward.

2 Breathing out, pull back your abdominal muscles to support your spine and, bending your knees, drop into a squat. This is great for building leg strength for labor. Reach out and grasp the object without hunching your back or shoulders. Make sure you have a firm grip and pull it toward your chest.

3 Pull up your pelvic floor muscles, breathe in and push into your heels to straighten your legs. Try to keep your back straight and the object clasped close to your body.

4 Before carrying the load, make sure the way ahead of you is clear, then keep the object close to your body. To put it down, stand directly in front of the new spot rather than twisting or turning, and squat as before. Make sure the load is firmly set on the spot before releasing your grip. Then push through your heels to come back to a standing position.

During pregnancy, limit the amount of weight you carry—try not to lift anything heavier than 11 lb, reducing this to around 4 lb by the third trimester. Therefore, you are limited to small bags of compost and banned from moving large containers, sacks of mulch, and wheelbarrows of manure. From the second trimester, make sure you are sitting down when you lift to avoid lightheadedness.

Before you start any lifting or carrying, make sure your body is well warmed-up—in one study this cut the risk of injury by almost one third. It's especially important to warm up if you are a weekend gardener, and stay mostly sedentary during weekdays.

CHOOSING THE RIGHT EQUIPMENT

Having a light spade or fork that fits your stature cuts the amount of effort you have to put into digging.

SPADES AND FORKS

While shorter spades and forks offer greater maneuverability, you may find it easier while pregnant to work with a longer handle, which prevents stooping. When you stand upright, the handle should reach your waist. If you're petite, you may find the more compact "border" fork or spade fits you better and is also easier when working in confined spaces, for instance when between rows of vegetables.

If you can't lift the spade without holding your breath when it doesn't have earth on it, you'll struggle in the garden, so look for the lightest quality tool.

Though they are more expensive, stainless steel heads require less maintenance: the soil glides off the blade, so you don't need to bend down to clean and oil it.

The shaft is the long piece of wood, plastic, or steel connecting the head and handle. A thicker shaft is easier to grip; you may find those made for disabled gardeners suit you if you suffer from carpal tunnel syndrome or swelling at the wrists.

You'll have more purchase on the tool if your foot fits comfortably on the top of the head, so check that the top is flat and wide enough to accommodate your gardening boots.

If you prefer a "D"-shaped top, check that your gloved hands fit easily within the handle.

A blade which is pointed at the bottom is good for digging holes, turning soil, and lifting plants; this is usually called a spade. A broader blade with only slight curves at the bottom and scooped edges—a shovel —is best for lifting and moving soil and other loose material (the curves keep the load in).

A sharp blade cuts through heavy soil and turf more effectively, and you can also use it to slice through roots and skim weeds from the surface (so you don't have to get down on hands and knees to pull them out). It's safest during pregnancy to have an expert sharpen your tools, rather than wielding clamps, steel wool, and files yourself.

To ease your workload, break up compacted or heavy soil with a fork before digging with a spade or shovel; for organic gardeners this has the added benefit of preserving the lives of worms. Because a fork doesn't allow you to exert the same amount of force as a spade, this is probably the safest way to loosen and turn soil and dig out plants.

A four-tined fork tends to make digging easier; it may be called a "spading fork."

WHEELBARROWS

The lighter the barrow the better during pregnancy, so if your current one is a builder-style galvanized metal model, treat yourself to a plastic version. While your balance is slightly off, choose a barrow with thick tires (inflatable ones are easy to maneuver) or a ball, for increased stability. To make the load even more stable, position the bulk of it over the wheel rather than near the handles. If the barrow ever seems about to topple, step back and allow it to fall. This is safer for you than trying to catch it awkwardly.

Instead of trying to heft heavy objects into a wheelbarrow, roll them onto a tarpaulin. Step in front of it, draw together the four corners, and drag the load behind you.

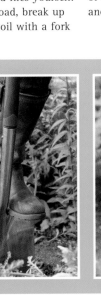
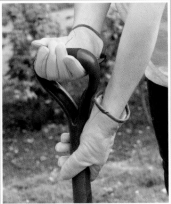
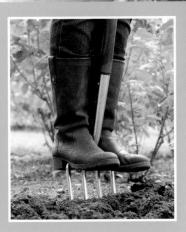

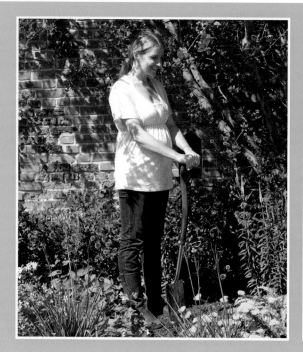
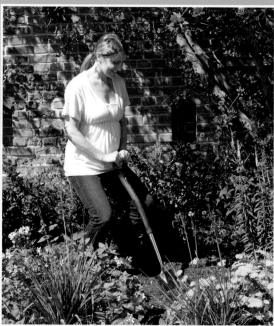

WORKING IN THE GARDEN

Once you've warmed up, aim at keeping your level of activity light to moderate—you should be able to talk even while working on the heaviest of gardening tasks. And keep breathing—it's temping to hold the breath when lifting, but you need to keep oxygen flowing to your baby.

Don't try to cram all your heavy tasks into a couple of hours—try to intersperse them with lighter work, such as weeding or deadheading. Doing one task for a concentrated period of time can lead to repetitive injuries, so aim for just 10 minutes on each, and have a good stretch and a short rest before moving on.

Divide tasks into a series of mini activities; if you have to move a number of containers, for example, shift them one by one rather than stacked, and remove the soil first. More trips with less weight is always safest—think of it as a gym workout with more repetitions of lighter weights. This is the best way to build the stamina you need to get through labor and delivery.

If you can't raise everything from seed this year, buy in young plug plants—you can get an entire kitchen garden shipped in this way.

After a gardening session, stretch out the muscles you have been working—after clipping, for example, stretch your arms wide and bend your wrists forward and back.

After digging (see below), stretch out your calves and thigh muscles.

Relax in the garden regularly to maintain peace of mind. Making space for a rocking seat or hammock now (fix permanent points to walls or posts) will pay dividends when you have babies and toddlers.

DIGGING

Old-fashioned gardeners swear by double-digging—lifting two spades' depths of soil and dumping them in two trenches—over single digging—moving only one spade's depth to one new trench. They say it gives better drainage and soil structure and blitzes stubborn weeds.

However, during pregnancy it's best not to over-tire yourself. Don't try to extend the amount of time you spend gardening or the strenuousness of the work. If you're used to gardening, opt for single digging, or for these few precious months turn to the even less strenuous simple digging—just lift one spade's depth of soil and put it back in the same position.

To avoid stressing your body, focus your attention on the muscles in your arms and legs while digging. This helps to protect your spine and abdomen.

1 Stand directly in front of the patch you are digging with feet hip-width apart. Place the blade on the top of the soil close to your body and parallel to the front of your feet. Make sure it's at a 90° angle to the ground.

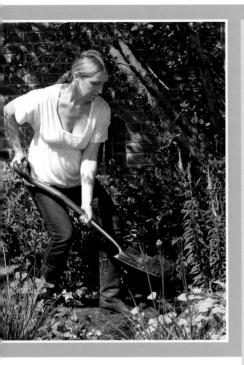

MAKING A RAISED BED

If you are growing your own vegetables during pregnancy, raised beds are by far the easiest option. They cut down on weeding and, perhaps more importantly, raise the ground level toward you, thus requiring less bending. The system also suits gardeners with very heavy soil or poor drainage. As an added extra, after construction you need never dig again; just add a new layer of compost to the top each year.

Ask someone else do the heavy work: maneuvering planks, heavy digging, and lifting or emptying bags of manure. Railroad ties make the quickest raised beds (no nails), but many are treated with wood preservatives that are not safe during pregnancy and could leach into food. Choose pressure-treated wood instead.

1 Measure out the size of the bed. Try one or two ties in length, and don't make it so wide than you can't comfortably reach halfway across. Mark out the area using string attached to pegs to give a straight line. Then mark the line with a spray can to avoid having to bend over.

2 Dig over the ground, being careful about your posture and overheating. Get someone else to lift turf and dig out large plants or deep-rooted weeds.

2 Step one foot onto the top of the blade, keeping your back straight and both hands on the handle. Press down using your top foot.

3 Keeping your back straight and chest wide, bend your arms and knees to position the soil on the blade. Try not to hold your breath.

4 To move the soil, slide one hand halfway down the shaft. Breathe out, pull your pelvic floor muscles in and your abdominal muscles toward your back, then lift the load. Keeping the load close to your body, pivot on one foot to move it, keeping the spade in front of you rather than twisting your spine. Bend your knees to lower the load.

3 Have the ties maneuvered into place over the marked lines. Make sure you're happy with the positioning before the workers leave.

4 On heavy soil, start by filling the new bed with a layer of gravel and sharp sand. Then add a mix of topsoil and compost, such as kitchen compost, well-rotted manure, leaf mold, or seaweed. As before, get someone else do the lifting, carrying, and pouring. Rake to a fine tilth and water well, ready to start sowing. When working at the bed, use a well-padded kneeler and face directly forward.

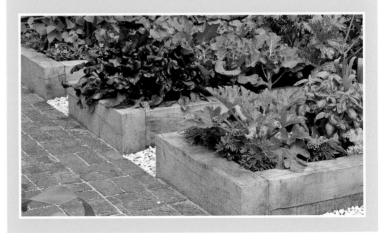

working in the garden

INDEX

ACKNOWLEDGMENTS

Most thanks of all to my husband, Stephen Parker, the brains of the garden and the master of the kitchen and range, for all his digging, seaweed mulching, obsessing about blight and triumphs in the raised beds and cooking pots.

To Ruth Cicale, special thanks for the sourdough starter and advice on getting the dough to rise.

Thanks also to Georgia Sawers for the best hummus, and to my father-in-law for his secret steak recipe.

Thanks, as always, to Amy Carroll for her inspiration and to Chrissie Lloyd for her designs. Also to Tracy Stewart-Murray and David Murray.

Carroll & Brown would like to thank:

Additional Art Direction Tracy Stewart-Murray
Home Economist Clare Lewis
IT Management John Casey

Picture Credits:
All images © Carroll & Brown with the exception of the following from Photolibrary.com:
p2, p12 background, p19 main, p22, p26, p32, p35, p48 background, center, p54 background, center, p62 background, p64, p68 main, p69, p74 background, center, p86 top, p87 right, p90 main, p92 center, p125 right

Bibliography

Pregnancy:
Having Faith: an ecologist's journey to motherhood, *Sandra Steingraber* (Berkley 2001)
Spiritual Midwifery, *Ina May Gaskin* (Book Publishing Company 2002)
Wise Woman Herbal for the Childbearing Year, *Susun S. Weed* (Ash Tree Publishing 1985)

Gardening:
The New Kitchen Garden, *Anna Pavord* (Dorling Kindersley 1999)
Grow Your Own Vegetables, *Joy Larkcom* (Frances Lincoln 2002)
Second Nature, a Gardener's Education, *Michael Pollan* (Grove Press 2003)

Food:
The River Cottage Meat Book, *Hugh Fearnley-Whittingstall* (Hodder and Stoughton 2004)
The River Cottage Fish Book, *Hugh Fearnley-Whittingstall* (Bloomsbury 2007)
Four Seasons Cookery Book, *Margaret Costa* (Grub Street 2008)
Moro East, *Sam and Sam Clark* (an allotment cookbook) (Ebury 2007)
Colin Spencer's Vegetable Book (Conran Octopus 1995)
A New Book of Middle Eastern Food, *Claudia Roden* (Penguin 1986)
Cooking with my Indian Mother-in-law, *Simon Daley with Roshan Hirani* (Pavilion, 2008)
The Italian Cookery Course, *Katie Caldesi* (Kyle Cathie 2009)
Roast Chicken and Other Stories, *Simon Hopkinson* (Ebury 1994)
Farmhouse Fare, recipes from Country Housewives collected by The Farmers Weekly (Countrywise Books 1966)